Matching Pursuit and Unification in EEG Analysis

This book is part of the
Artech House Engineering in Medicine and Biology Series,
Martin L. Yarmush and Christopher J. James, Series Editors.
For a list of recent related Artech House titles,
please turn to the back of this book.

Matching Pursuit and Unification in EEG Analysis

Piotr Durka

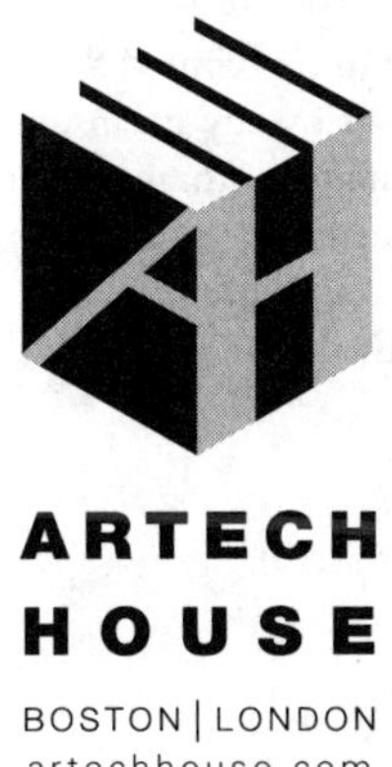

ARTECH HOUSE
BOSTON | LONDON
artechhouse.com

Library of Congress Cataloging-in-Publication Data
A catalog record for this book is available from the U.S. Library of Congress.

British Library Cataloguing in Publication Data
A catalogue record for this book is available from the British Library.

ISBN 13: 978-1-58053-304-1

Cover design by Igor Valdman

685 Canton Street
Norwood, MA 02062

10 9 8 7 6 5 4 3 2 1

Contents

Foreword

Piotr Durka has written an unusual book on the analysis of the electroencephalogram (EEG) that goes beyond the mathematical fundaments and the subtleties of signal analysis. He proposes an original "unifying theory" that may account for how different aspects of EEG signals may be analyzed within a common theoretical framework.

This is an ambitious objective. He shows in this book how this objective may be achieved in clear language, for specialists in signal analysis and clinical neurophysiologists alike. The studies on which this book is based stem from the research line pursued in the course of the last decades by the Warsaw group led by Katarzyna Blinowska. This book represents a comprehensive account of the theoretical and mathematical basis of adaptive time-frequency EEG signal analysis, as well as of the methodology of how the corresponding algorithms can be implemented in everyday practice.

This book represents a novel link between the visually guided feature extraction approach made by the electroencephalographer in everyday practice, and the advanced computer analysis based on "matching pursuit" and related algorithms. In this way, this book provides a remarkable synthesis between theory and practice. This important contribution to the literature should be an incentive to advance the field of electroencephalography, both for theoreticians and clinical neurophysiologists.

Fernando Lopes da Silva, M.D., Ph.D.
University of Amsterdam
Amsterdam, the Netherlands
March 2007

Preface

The widespread availability of powerful personal computers gives a new meaning to the term *applied* signal processing. Advanced methods are becoming available to users with little mathematical background. Among these methods, adaptive time-frequency approximations of signals are special in more than one respect:

- They unify many desired properties of previously applied methods, such as high time-frequency resolution, sparse representations, explicit parameterization of transients, and adaptivity, which offers freedom from prior settings.
- Under the hood, there is advanced mathematics, yet the output is intuitive and easy to interpret.
- Known algorithms—implementations of the matching pursuit (MP)—are computer-intensive. This inhibited their practical applications before the last decade, but today they can run on a standard PC.

Signal processing cannot exist without the context of real-world applications. We choose a fascinating context: recordings of the electrical activity of the human brain—the electroencephalogram (EEG). For more than 70 years, EEG have been the most direct trace of thought that we can measure. Recently, electroencephalography seems to have lost importance in favor of new brain imaging techniques—in spite of their only indirect relation to the neuronal signaling, low time resolution, and high cost. Why? Magnetic resonance imaging and positron emission tomography offer results in terms of easily interpretable, computed images; no clinician or neurophysiologist would use the raw signals recorded by the sensors. Funny as it may sound, visual analysis of raw EEG recordings is still the state of the art in clinical electroencephalography—basically unchanged in 70 years.

This book gives blueprints to bridge the gap between the tradition of visual EEG analysis and advanced signal processing. From the same basic ideas, we also derive complete frameworks that open new possibilities in several research paradigms: classical and continuous descriptions of sleep recordings (polysomnograms), microstructure of event-related EEG desynchronization and synchronization, detection/description of epileptic spikes and seizures, pharmaco EEG, and source localization (preprocessing for EEG inverse solutions). The sum of these applications suggests that presented paradigms can unify at least some elements of the art of visual EEG interpretation with advanced signal processing. They also unify advantages of different signal processing methods applied previously in this field. Such common methodological framework may significantly improve the reliability of both clinical and research applications of EEG.

Contents of This Book

Digital revolution opens amazing possibilities, but computers do not think for us. To be responsible for the results, we must understand what we are doing. In biomedical sciences, "we" cannot relate only to mathematicians and engineers. Therefore, the first part of this book gives a minimal necessary background in signal processing, using only plain English and no equations. Starting from basic notions like sampling of analog signals, inner product, orthogonality, and uncertainty principle, through spectral and time-frequency methods of signal analysis (spectrogram and wavelets), we arrive at the idea of adaptive approximations and the basics of the matching pursuit algorithm. Chapters 6 and 7 summarize major advantages and caveats related to its applications, with references to examples from Part II.

Each of the applications presented in Part II explores some particular and unique feature of the matching pursuit. Starting from the explicit parameterization of signal structures in terms of their amplitudes, time widths and time and frequency centers, through high-resolution and robust estimates of time-frequency energy density and their averages in event-related paradigms, to selective estimates of the energy of relevant structures, which improve the sensitivity of pharmaco-EEG and stability of EEG inverse solutions. Similar to Part I, these presentations are basically equation-free. Software used in these studies is freely available from http://eeg.pl. For the mathematically oriented readers, Part III introduces formally adaptive approximations and related technical issues, including the mathematical tricks necessary in efficient implementations of the matching pursuit algorithm.

Part I

Some Basic Notions

Chapter 1

Signal: Going Digital

This chapter discusses some basic laws of the digital world relevant to the discrete representation of analog signals.

A signal carries information. In the digital era, information is expressed by numbers. For some kinds of information, like school grades, stock values, or written texts,[1] digital representation is natural and direct. Other signals are continuous and analog by their nature—like sound. What we hear reflects the continuous changes of air density. In the predigital, analog era, we used to record these changes on magnetic tapes by converting the motion of a microphone's membrane into variable magnetization. To play back recorded sounds, we drove membranes of loudspeakers with an amplified electric current, reproducing directly the magnetization pattern stored on the tape.

Nowadays, in between the recording and playback, we introduce additional steps: the analog-digital conversion (A/D)—that is converting the signal to a sequence of numbers—and the inverse, digital-analog conversion (D/A), for playback. These stages are ever-present—in recording and reproducing music, videos, and biomedical signals. Before going any further, we consider consequences of the digital storage and processing of signals.

1 If we assign a number to each letter (best according to the ASCII or UNICODE standards), books and poems become sequences of numbers.

1.1 SAMPLING

To store an analog signal in the digital form (i.e., as a sequence of numbers), we measure its values in a series of time instants. Measurements are usually equally spaced in time—by a constant *sampling interval.* Reciprocal of the sampling interval is the sampling frequency, that is the number of samples per second (in Hz).

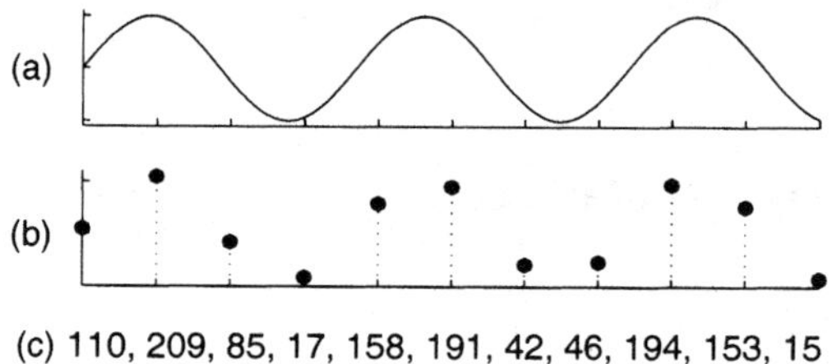

Figure 1.1 (a) Continuous signal, (b) its values at the sampling points, and (c) stored numbers (i.e., digital representation of the signal).

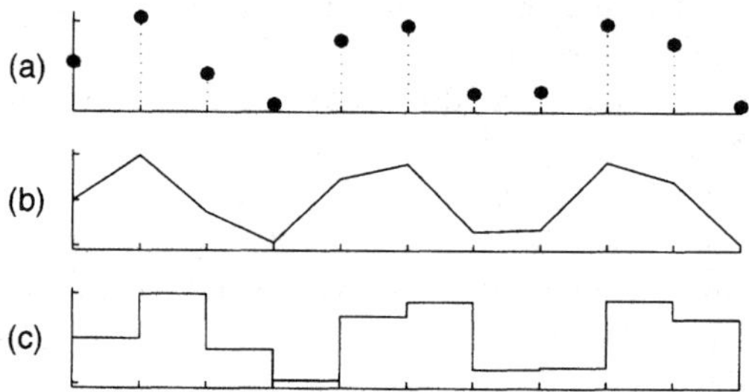

Figure 1.2 (b), (c) Possible reconstructions of the signal (a), sampled in Figure 1.1.

Sampling converts a continuous signal—Figure 1.1(a)—into a sequence of numbers (c). To play back the sound stored in this form on a CD, we must reconstruct from this sequence an analog signal to drive the amplifier. That requires filling in the empty spaces between measurements. But how do we recover the values in between? Figure 1.2 gives some simple "guesses," but if we compare them to the original signal from Figure 1.1, it is obvious that none of them is correct.

So, do we lose a lot of information here? Should we retract all the praises of the CD quality? Fortunately it's not that bad. If the analog signal (before sampling) fulfills certain conditions (in relation to the sampling frequency), we can even reconstruct the analog signal *exactly* from the stored numbers. Roughly, these assumptions say that the signal cannot fluctuate (oscillate) too much compared to the sampling interval.

Obviously, the signal should not oscillate between the samples, because then we would be unable to reconstruct or analyze the variability, occurring between the samples, from the digital representation—these details would be lost. But is that all?

1.2 DRAWBACK: ALIASING

The upper plot of Figure 1.3 presents a signal, sampled with an obviously too low frequency.[2] In the sequence of samples (black dots), significant details are missing: entire humps of the sine wave occur in between the sampling points, and there is no way to guess their presence from the digital sequence after such sampling.

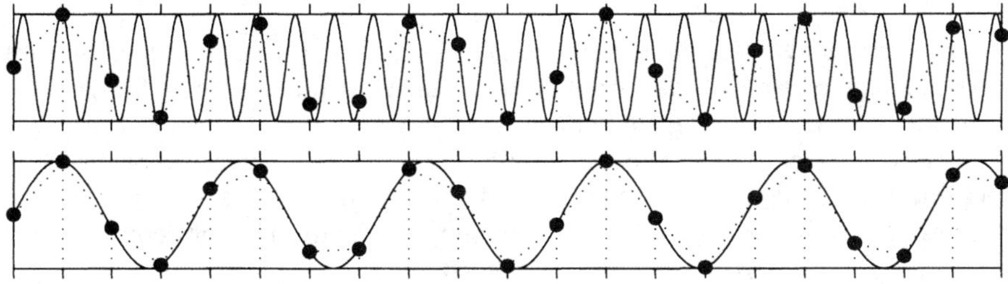

Figure 1.3 Two analog sine waves sampled with the same frequency. Black dots denote stored values.

However, if we compare closely two sequences resulting from sampling the two different signals presented in the lower and upper plots, we notice that the situation is much worse than that. Not only do we lose some information, but the higher frequency signal (upper plot) in its sampled version is indistinguishable from the sequence resulting from sampling a certain lower frequency signal (lower plot). Therefore, in a signal containing both these frequencies, lower frequency components of the sampled signal will be significantly distorted by false contributions from the higher, improperly sampled frequencies.

How dense do we have to sample analog signals to avoid such distortion and loss of information? If a reasonable relation is kept between the sampling frequency and the maximum frequencies of the sampled waves, like in the lower panel of

2 Or, saying the same the other way, containing frequencies too high for the chosen sampling interval.

Figure 1.3, then we should be able to reconstruct the original wave with good accuracy.

Figure 1.4 presents sampling of few waves, oscillating at frequencies close to the sampling frequency. We can imagine the information content of the sequence of numbers (digital signal) as only the black dots. Looking at these dots only, in some cases we cannot guess that in the analog signal from which these samples were taken, some higher frequency was present. Oscillations above half of the sampling frequency are irrecoverable from the sampled signals. As for the waves below half the sampling frequency, digital sequences seems to carry enough information for their reconstruction. These empirical results are in perfect agreement with the Nyquist-Shannon theorem, which says:

> When sampling a signal, the sampling frequency must be greater than twice the bandwidth of the input signal in order to be able to reconstruct the original perfectly from the sampled version.

This theorem is also known as the Whittaker-Nyquist-Kotelnikov-Shannon sampling theorem or simply the sampling theorem. Half the sampling frequency is sometimes called the Nyquist frequency.

How do we retrieve the amplitude of the analog signal in between the samples? The solution (which requires a bit of mathematics) is quite different from the guesses sketched in Figure 1.2. Correct interpolation formula relies on the "sinc" function ($\text{sinc}(x) = \frac{\sin(x)}{x}$), which looks like this:

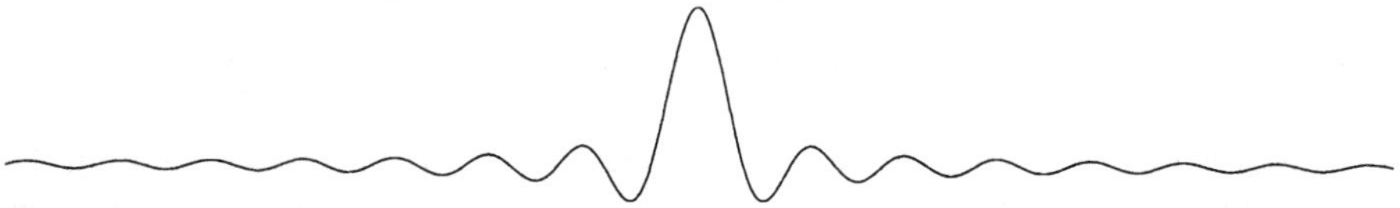

If we place one such function in each of the sampled points, with amplitude given by the value in that point, and add them all up, we recover the original, continuous signal.

But we have to remember that the derivation of the sampling theorem is based upon a very strong assumption—that the sampled signal is perfectly band-limited (i.e., there are no frequencies above half the sampling frequency). If this assumption is not fulfilled, digital/analog conversion will give a signal that may significantly differ from the original. And the differences will *not* be limited to high frequencies—due to an improper sampling, low frequencies will also be distorted. Therefore, analysis of such an improperly sampled sequence will give erroneous results.

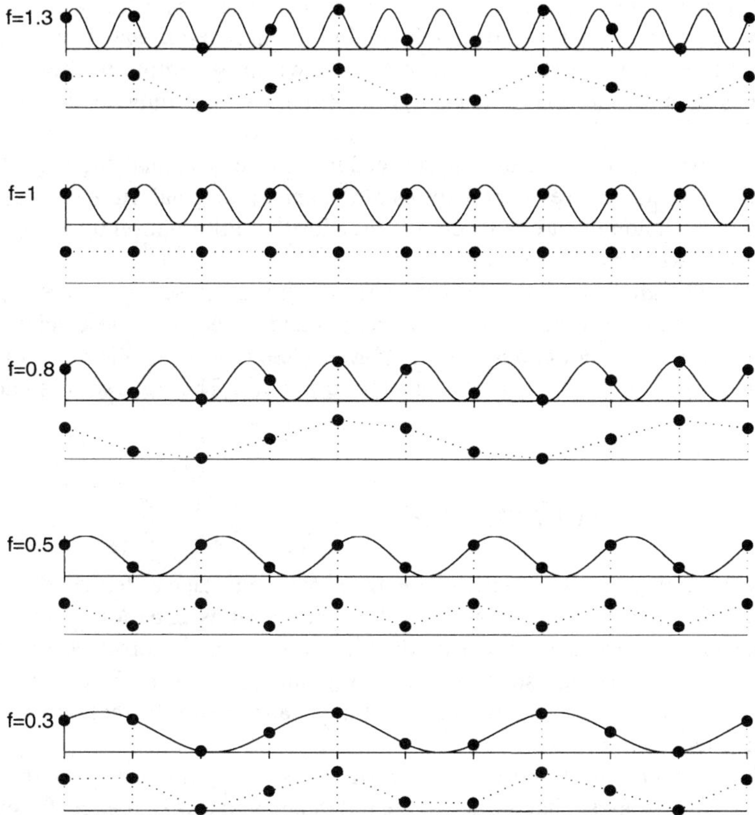

Figure 1.4 Analog, continuous waves of different frequencies, sampled (digitized) with the same unit frequency—for example 1 Hz or 1 kHz (in these cases, the sampling interval would be one second and one millisecond, correspondingly). For the sine wave of frequency f=0.3, shown in the lower panel, reproduction of the original frequency of oscillations from the digitized sequence seems possible. Half of the sampling frequency (f=0.5) is a border case: per each period of the wave, we get two samples, making it still possible to mark both the humps (positive and negative) occurring in one period. Higher frequencies, presented in the upper three panels, cannot be reproduced from the sampled sequence. The specific case of a frequency exactly equal to the sampling frequency (f=1) results in a flat digital representation—a loss of information but still no distortion. In the other cases, exemplified by f=0.8 and f=1.3, sampling these high frequencies produces a digital signal from which we *falsely* read the presence of some lower frequencies. This effect is stressed in Figure 1.3.

In practice we can seldom assume that a given signal is perfectly band-limited. Therefore, prior to sampling we apply analog *antialiasing filters*. For example, if we are interested in frequencies up to 50 Hz, we must sample the signal with a frequency of at least 100 Hz, and prior to sampling we must remove the oscillations above 50 Hz.[3]

Properly performed sampling procedures can ensure that the digital signal will reliably reflect the relevant features of the analog original. In plain English we can say that if enough care is taken, we may lose no information by going digital. But what do we earn?

Digital signals can be analyzed using general purpose computers: new processing algorithms can be easily implemented and tested. But these scientific applications are surely not enough reason for all the everyday applications of digital technology—such as CDs, DVDs, or mobile phones. There must be some other profits.

1.3 ADVANTAGE: CHECKSUMS

Quality of analog sound or video, stored on magnetic tapes, degrades with time and use. Every copy incorporates all the nonlinearities and noise produced by each player and recorder. Similarly, damages on vinyl LPs produce sounds that cannot be a priori distinguished from their original content.[4] On the contrary, in the digital world we can achieve perfection of any transfer of information—including copying—using *checksums*.

After sampling (Figure 1.1), the signal is represented by a sequence of numbers. Now suppose that we add some redundancy to this sequence, for example by placing, after every seven numbers, the eighth one as their sum—the checksum. This is excess information, since instead of sending (copying) the whole redundant sequence, its every eighth number can be easily reproduced after receiving or reading the preceeding seven. However, if we receive or read the whole sequence including checksums, we can independently calculate the sum of every seven numbers and compare it with the eighth (the checksum) that we have read or received. If they do not match, we know that the sequence was distorted during

3 Online analog filters are unable to exactly "cut" all oscillations above a certain frequency, so the low-pass attenuation usually starts at a frequency lower than the critical half of the sampling frequency. Therefore, we should actually sample signals at least slightly above the (doubled) highest frequency of interest.

4 Sophisticated signal processing techniques can be developed to partially restore the original sound, but they are far from automatic and must be carefully supervised.

transfering or copying. However, in this simple example the contrary does not hold (i.e., if the checksum verifies OK, there may be, for example, two equal errors of opposite sign). Therefore, more sophisticated checksum algorithms are implemented for applications.

What can we do with this knowledge? Depending on the situation, there are different possibilities:

- If the error occurred during transfer, we (that is, the computer program in control of the transfer) may simply ask the sender to resend the corrupted part, until the checksum verifies OK. This is why Internet packets contain the addresses of both the sender and receiver.
- The same procedure applies to copying—using checksums, we can verify the accuracy of the copy and proceed similarly if the distortion occurred during the transfer from the original.
- If we discover that part of the data is corrupted, knowing it is always superior to ignorance:
  - In real systems, redundancy is introduced in an intelligent way, allowing the use of the extra information for the recovery of distorted parts. The idea can be imagined as two copies of the same song stored on a CD: if a part of the major copy reveals a checksum error, the device plays the corresponding part from the second copy.
  - Even if there is no way to recover the original content, still "it's good to know." For example, it is better if a CD player plays nothing rather than a false crash, which may result from a distortion of a few samples. "Nothing" happening in a few samples of CD music will most likely pass unheard, since there are 44,100 samples per second. Silence in a few of them will be filtered out by the inertion of the loudspeakers.

Sophisticated techniques, based upon these simple ideas, allow for an error-free copy and transfer of digital data, and intelligent error handling in case of failures.

Chapter 2

Analysis

We introduce the notions of inner product, orthogonality, frequency, and phase.

An analysis is a critical evaluation, usually made by breaking a subject (either material or intellectual) down into its constituent parts, then describing the parts and their relationship to the whole.[1] Signal analysis usually consists of breaking the signal down into known functions. Different methods of analysis rely on different sets of "known" functions—we shall call these sets *dictionaries*.

To find out which of the functions best explain a given signal, we need a measure of fit (similarity) between the analyzed signal and a known function. Effectively, we need to measure similarity between two signals.

2.1 INNER PRODUCT—A MEASURE OF FIT

The most widely used measure of similarity between two signals is their inner product. Just like the product of two numbers, the inner product of two signals is a single number. How do we calculate it? We could multiply the value in each point of the first signal by the corresponding value of the second signal—but then we would be left with as many products as there were points. So we simply add them up.

1 http://en.wikipedia.org/wiki/Analysis.

For example, let us take two signals x and y as:

$$x = (2, 2, -2, 1, 2)$$
$$y = (-1, -1, 1, 1, 0)$$

their inner product is

$$x \cdot y = 2 \cdot (-1) + 2 \cdot (-1) + (-2) \cdot 1 + 1 \cdot 1 + 2 \cdot 0 = -5.$$

We may visualize this by putting one sequence above the other:

x	2	2	−2	1	2	
y	−1	−1	1	1	0	
$\cdot$	−2	−2	−2	1	0	$x \cdot y = -5$

Graphical representation of this operation (and signals) looks like this:

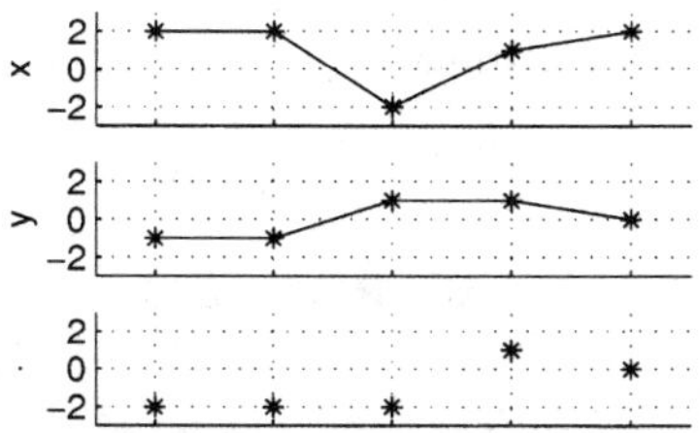

Signal in the lowest plot contains, in each sample, the product of the corresponding samples of the input signals x and y. The sum of the samples of this signal gives the inner product of the input signals $x \cdot y$. In this case the inner product is negative, because positive values of the first signal occur mostly in the points, where the samples of the second signal are negative, and vice versa. These signals do not fit each other, which implies a relatively low value of the inner product.

If we replace the first signal by its negative $(-1) \cdot x$, the value of the inner product $x \cdot y$ jumps from -5 to 5. These two signals fit each other much better (i.e., higher values of x and y are more likely to occur in the same places) as presented in the following plot and table:

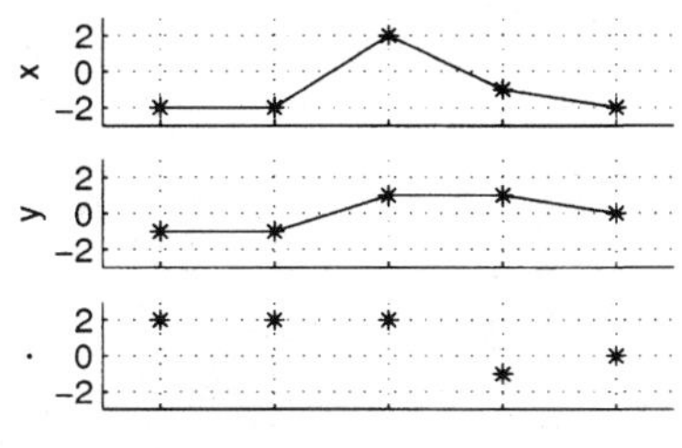

x	-2	-2	2	-1	-2	
y	-1	-1	1	1	0	
$\cdot$	2	2	2	-1	0	$x \cdot y = 5$

The best possible fit occurs in between the signal and itself.

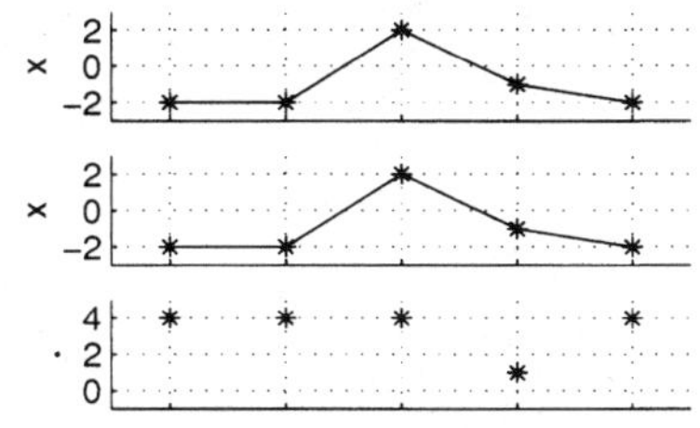

x	-2	-2	2	-1	-2	
x	-2	-2	2	-1	-2	
$\cdot$	4	4	4	1	4	$x \cdot x = 17$

Inner product $x \cdot x$, equivalent to the sum of the squares of all the values of x, gives in this case 17. This magnitude can be interpreted as the energy of the signal.

In general, if two signals are in phase[2] (i.e., maxima of one signal meet the maxima of the other signal), their product will be large:

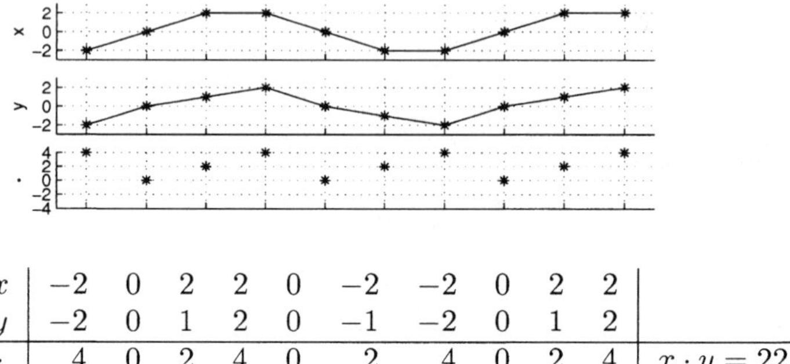

x	-2	0	2	2	0	-2	-2	0	2	2	
y	-2	0	1	2	0	-1	-2	0	1	2	
$\cdot$	4	0	2	4	0	2	4	0	2	4	$x \cdot y = 22$

But if we shift one of the signals so that its maxima approach the minima of the other signal (inverse phase), their inner product drops dramatically:

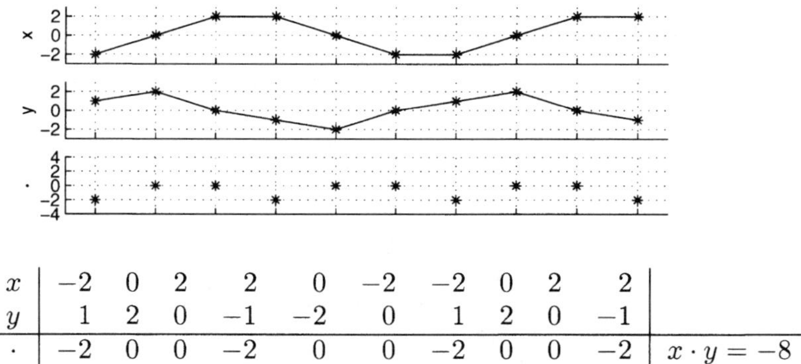

x	-2	0	2	2	0	-2	-2	0	2	2	
y	1	2	0	-1	-2	0	1	2	0	-1	
$\cdot$	-2	0	0	-2	0	0	-2	0	0	-2	$x \cdot y = -8$

These examples indicate that large values of the inner product indeed occur for similar signals; therefore, after solving some normalization problems,[3] we can use the inner product as a measure of similarity between two signals.

2 To give a large inner product, these signals should also have the same main frequency; frequency and phase will be discussed in Section 2.3.

3 The value of the inner product also depends on the magnitudes of signals, corresponding to the signal's energies (i.e., the products of the signals with themselves). When fitting known functions to a given signal, we take the vectors representing these functions so that they have a unit energy.

2.2 ORTHOGONALITY

For some pairs of signals, the inner product is zero; such signals are called orthogonal.

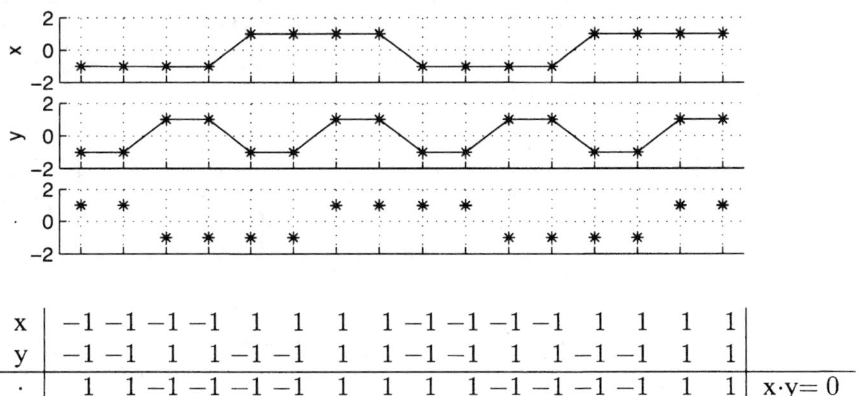

x	−1	−1	−1	−1	1	1	1	1	−1	−1	−1	−1	1	1	1	1	
y	−1	−1	1	1	−1	−1	1	1	−1	−1	1	1	−1	−1	1	1	
·	1	1	−1	−1	−1	−1	1	1	1	1	−1	−1	−1	−1	1	1	x·y= 0

In this example, the period of the lower signal is half of the period of the upper one. As an effect, half of the samples in each hump of the upper signal are multiplied by -1, and the other half by 1. The sum of these products will be zero if we add them on any whole number of periods (and at least one of the signals has a zero mean—both positive and negative values).

Dictionaries composed of functions that are mutually orthogonal are very convenient for the analysis of signals. The most popular one is formed from sine waves: any two sines of frequencies, that are integer multiples (harmonics) of a common base frequency, are mutually orthogonal (Figure 2.1).

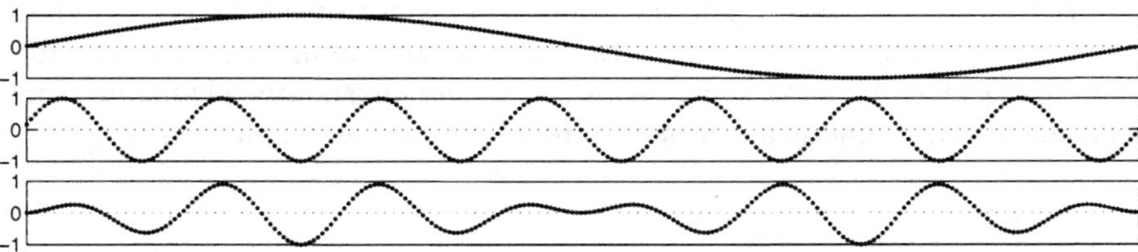

Figure 2.1 The second sine (middle plot) has a frequency seven times the frequency of the sine in the upper panel. Their product, point by point, is presented in the lower trace. The sum of all these point-by-point products—that is, the inner product of these signals—gives zero, so the vectors are orthogonal.

2.3 FREQUENCY AND PHASE

In plain English, frequency is the number of occurrences within a given time period[4]—for example for the frequency measured in Hertz (Hz), within 1 second.

In Figure 2.2, there are two equally spaced, identical rectangles in each second: we say that this rectangle wave has frequency 2 Hz. The wave in Figure 2.3 is composed of the same rectangles, occurring with the same frequency. What is the difference between them? *Phase*.

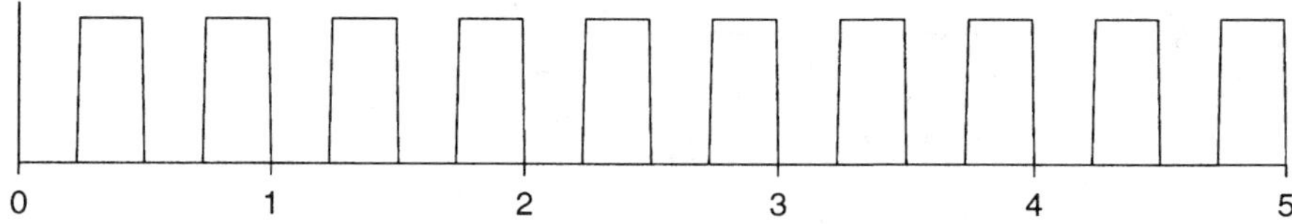

Figure 2.2 Rectangle wave of frequency 2 Hz (i.e., two humps per second).

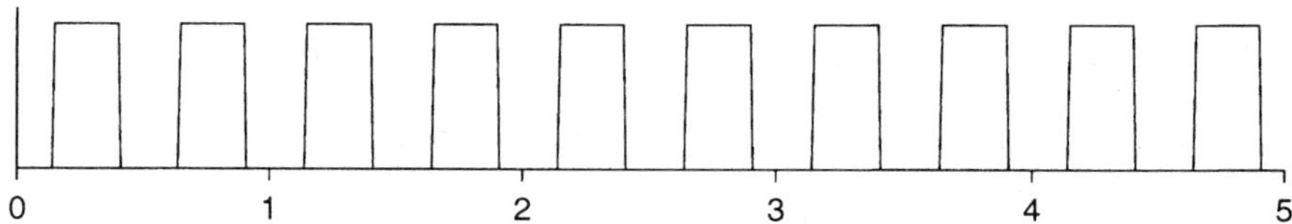

Figure 2.3 Another train of rectangles occurring, as in Figure 2.2, with frequency 2 Hz. However, in this signal, rectangles occur in different time points—obviously the starting point of the series was different than in Figure 2.2. We say that these signals differ in phase.

Phase is always relative to some point in time, but the difference of phases between two signals is an absolute value. It is usually measured in units of π, where 2π corresponds to a whole period. Shifting the phase of an infinite periodic signal by 2π gives exactly the same signal—it is called *phase ambiguity*: phase difference x is effectively the same as the phase difference $2\pi + x$, $4\pi + x$, and so on.

4 Period is the shortest distance between repeating parts of the signal; in Figure 2.2 it's 0.5 second. It is also the reciprocal of the frequency—and vice versa, the frequency is the reciprocal of the period.

The notion of phase is applicable to any periodic signal. Figure 2.4 presents two sine waves with the same frequency and different phases.

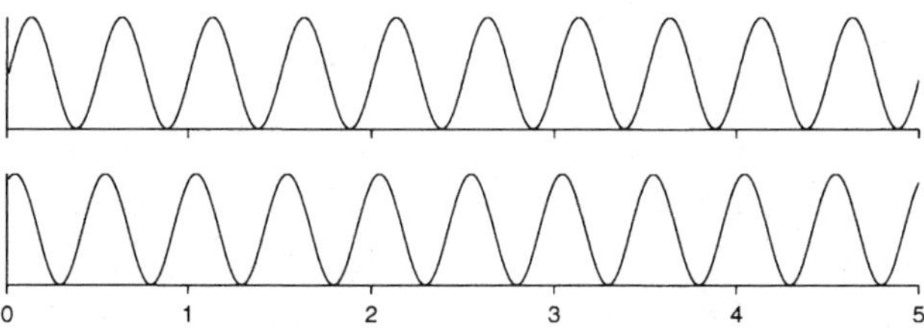

Figure 2.4 Two sines with the same frequency (2 Hz) and different phases.

If the humps of one signal do not occur in the same points as those of the other signal, this may be due to the different phases—but only if both signals have the same frequency. If the frequencies differ, the signals desynchronize, even if started with the same phase (Figure 2.5).

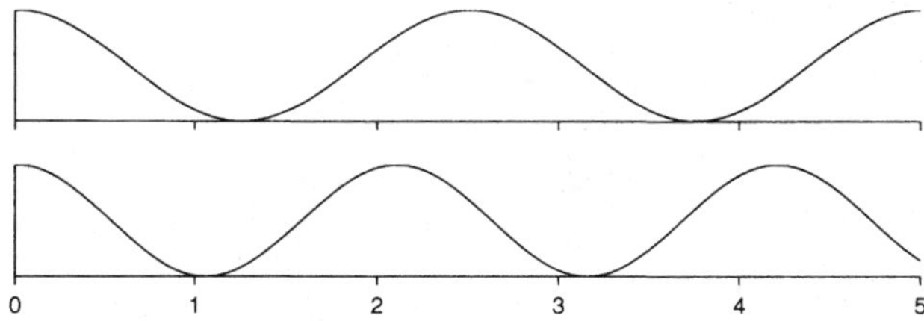

Figure 2.5 Two sines (upper and lower plot) starting with the same phase; due to different frequencies, their maxima desynchronize quickly.

Chapter 3

Spectrum

Using the basic notions of frequency, phase, and product explained in the previous chapter, this chapter addresses the meaning and estimation of energy spectrum.

Spectrum is the collection of the color rays of which light is composed; they can be separated by a prism. Similarly, a periodic signal (like the one in Figure 3.1) may contain several oscillations of different frequencies. How can we separate them and measure their content?

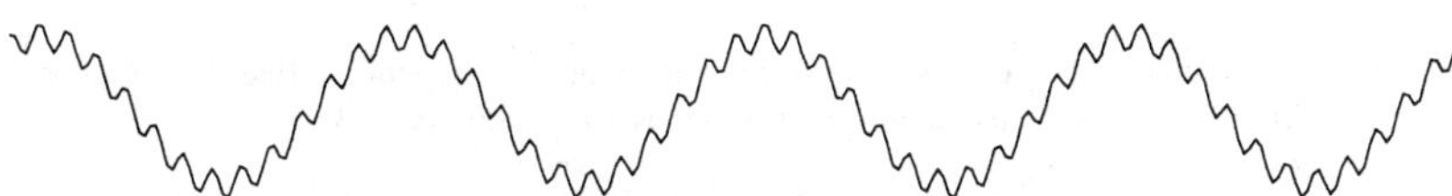

Figure 3.1 A signal containing two oscillations.

First of all, we need a template of "pure frequency." Once we choose the basic waveforms, we can measure the content of such "reference oscillations" in a given signal by means of the inner products with the signal.

Which of the infinite number of possible periodic waveforms should we take as the template? A sawtooth, sine, or maybe a square wave? Some possible candidates are presented in Figure 3.2.

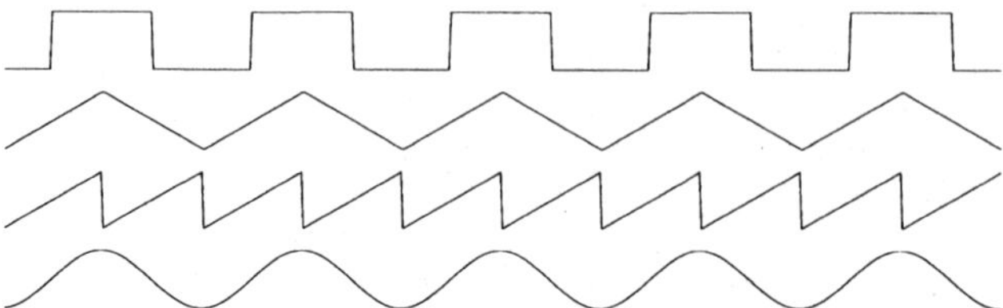

Figure 3.2 Some of the candidates for a template of "pure frequency" (from the top): square, triangle, sawtooth, and sinusoidal waveforms.

And the winner is ... sine!

Why sine? Actually, we could build some kind of frequency analysis using any periodic wave. But sine[1] is not only nice and smooth—it also passes unchanged through any linear time-invariant (LTI)[2] system. Why is this so important? LTI systems are the basis for the whole classical theory of signal processing. Decomposing a signal into building blocks, basic in terms of LTI systems, is advantageous in many situations.

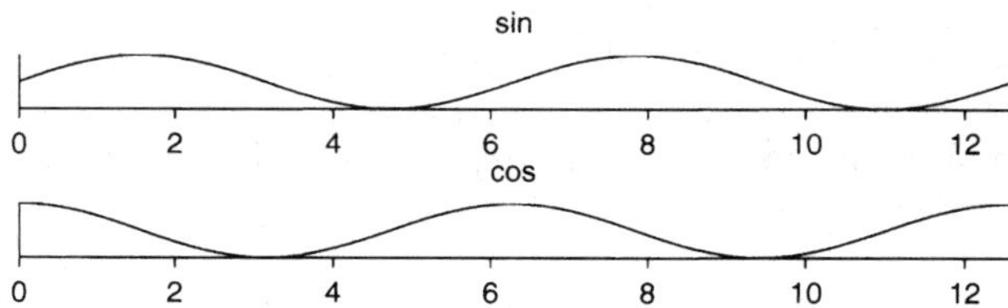

Figure 3.3 Sine (upper plot) and cosine (lower). The cosine is the sine shifted by a quarter of the period. The difference in phase between sine and cosine is 90 degrees or $\pi/4$.

1 Why sines, rather than cosines? Cosines share the same properties with regard to LTI systems. Actually, what's the difference between sine and cosine? As we see from Figure 3.3, cosine is a sine shifted by a quarter of the period (phase difference of 90 degrees or $\pi/4$). So which of them will better suit our needs? Oscillations present in the analyzed signal can have *any* phase—zero (sine), $\pi/4$ (cosine), or any other. Therefore, we must take into account all the possible phases. If we start with sines, cosines will come out as phase $\pi/4$. The classical Fourier expansion can be based on combinations of sines and cosines, since from their weighted sum we can reconstruct any phase.

2 Linearity and time invariance are reasonable requirements for many systems, also assumed in most of the digital signal processing (DSP) applications. For example, in case of an amplifier, the linearity means basically the lack of disturbances, and time invariance guarantees that the song played (amplified) in the morning will sound the same in the evening. "Unchanged" in this context means that a sine entering any LTI system comes out as a sine, with possibly changed amplitude and phase. For other waveforms, LTI systems change not only amplitude and phase, but also their shape.

3.1 EXAMPLE CALCULATIONS

Now that we have chosen the frequency template, we must find out which frequencies of the sines fit the analyzed signal. According to Section 2.1, we can measure this fit using the product of a sine of a given frequency with the signal. Now, we check the products of all possible sines with the signal and find those that fit best. A simplified view on the calculation of the spectrum may be summarized as follows:

1. We pick sine waves (Figure 3.4) with frequencies up to the half of the signal's sampling frequency (Nyquist frequency, Section 1.2).

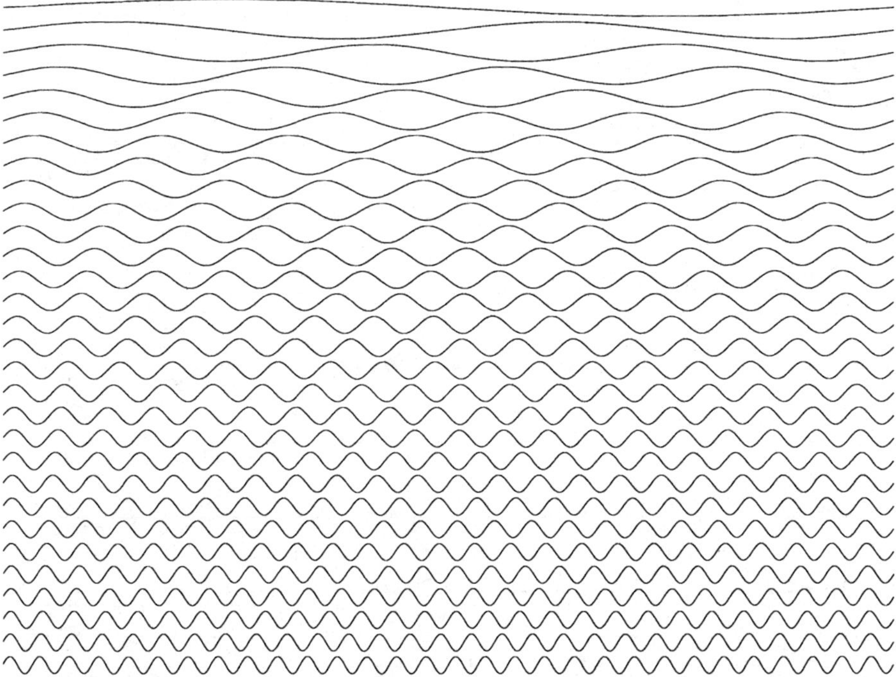

Figure 3.4 The first 30 sines from the dictionary used in Fourier transform. If the whole epoch lasts 1 second, then the first wave from the top has a frequency of 1 Hz, the second has a frequency of 2 Hz, and the lowest one, 30 Hz. All these signals are mutually orthogonal.

2. For each of these frequencies, we find the maximal product with the signal by trying different phases. This process is illustrated in Figure 3.5 for a single frequency. In practice, the choice of an optimal phase is effectuated by a mathematical trick using complex numbers.

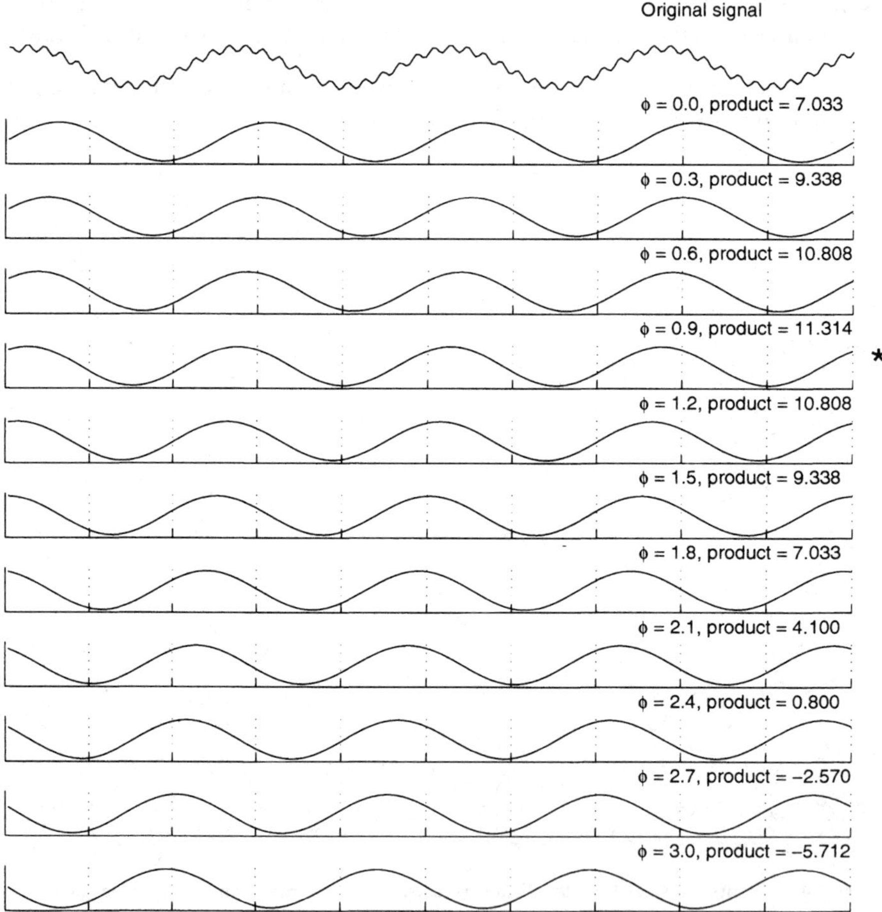

Figure 3.5 Finding the phase (ϕ) of a sine of a given frequency, maximizing its inner product with the signal. The sine with the optimal phase is marked by a star on the right.

3. Inner products of the signal with sines, for which optimal phases were found in the previous step, give us the contents of the signal's energy, carried by corresponding frequencies, as visualized in Figure 3.6.

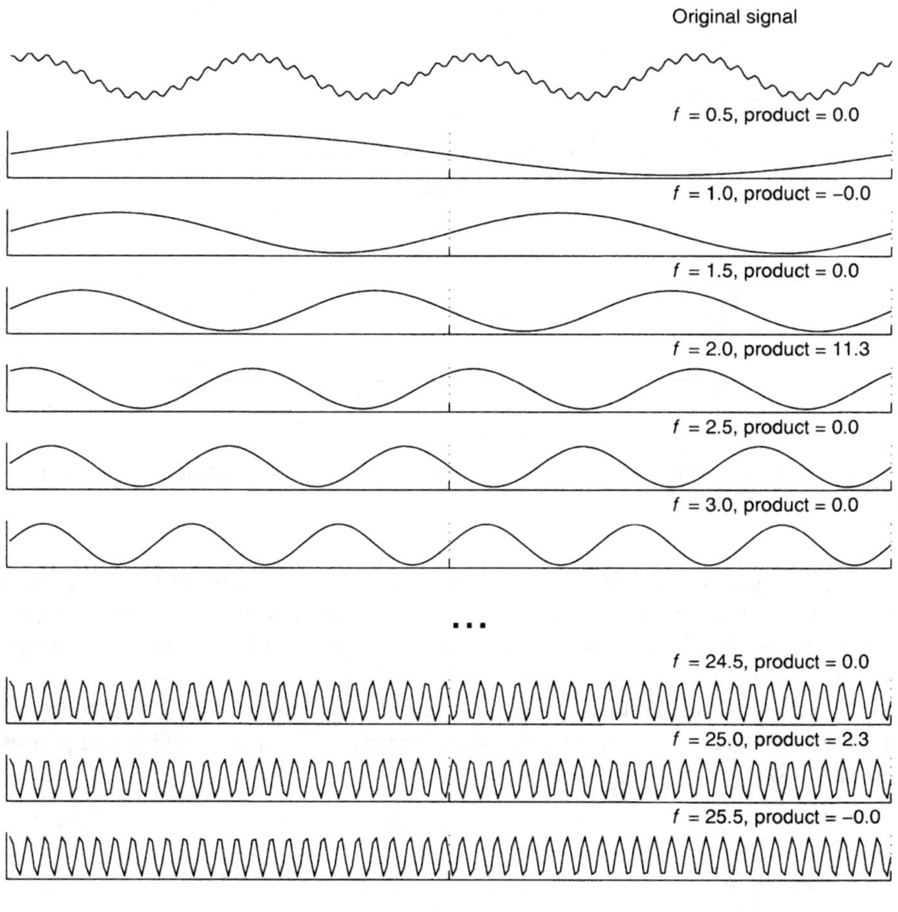

Figure 3.6 Products of sines with different frequencies (f), and phases optimized for each frequency in the previous step (Figure 3.5), with the signal.

As a result of this analysis, in Figure 3.7 we can plot the inner products of the sines with the signal and corresponding optimal phases (for nonzero products).

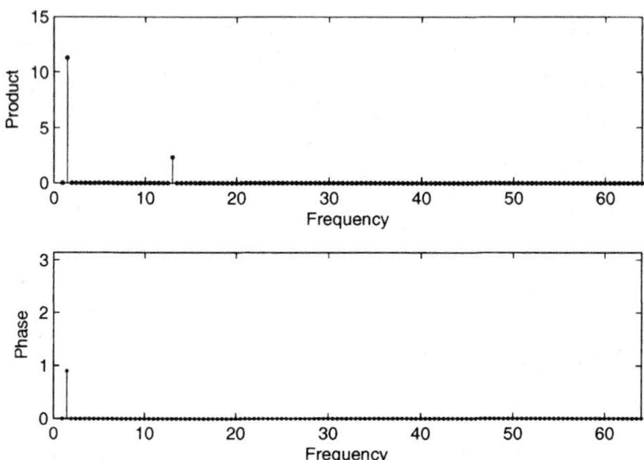

Figure 3.7 Results of the spectral analysis of the signal from Figure 3.1: upper panel—power spectrum; lower panel—phase spectrum.

In the upper panel of Figure 3.7, we observe that only two frequencies give nonzero products with the signal. Such perfectly clear results are obtained mainly for simulated signals; real-world spectra are much more complex and noisy, which will be discussed in the next section.

In any case, using the information presented in Figure 3.7, we can reconstruct the original signal as a sum of sines with properly chosen amplitudes and phases (Figure 3.8).

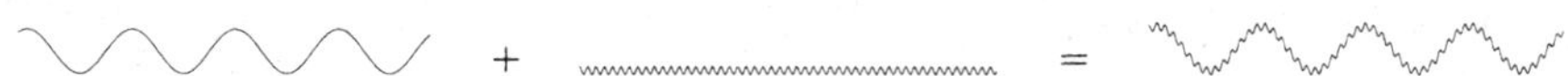

Figure 3.8 Reconstruction of the signal from Figure 3.1 using the products and phases presented in Figure 3.7.

The usual way of presenting the signal's power spectrum is just the upper panel of Figure 3.7, plotted with a continuous line as in Figure 3.9.

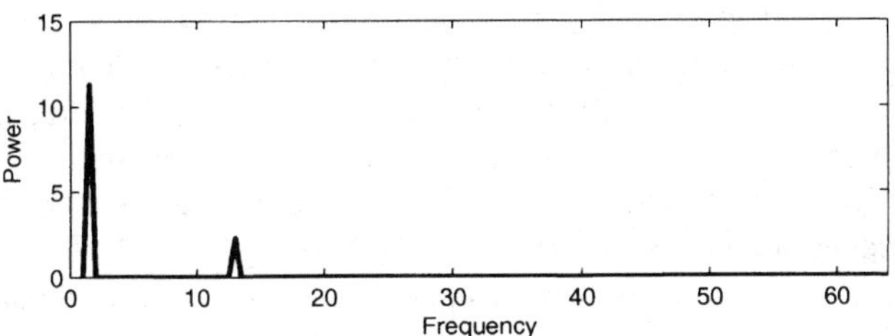

Figure 3.9 Power spectrum from the upper panel of Figure 3.7, plotted with a continuous line.

3.2 UNCERTAINTY PRINCIPLE AND RESOLUTION

According to the conclusions from Section 1.2, the frequency scale ends at the Nyquist frequency, which for the signal sampled at 128 Hz is 64 Hz. How many points do we have in this frequency range? If the numbers presented in Figure 3.7 exactly suffice to reconstruct the original signal, they should contain as much information as the signal itself. So let us look back at the signal in its raw form, as presented in Figure 3.10.

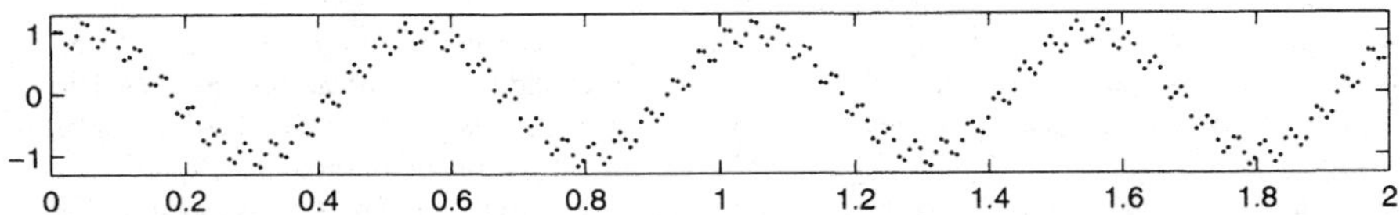

Figure 3.10 Exact representation of the digital signal presented in Figures 3.1, 3.5, and 3.6 as a continuous line connecting the samples. The 256 samples with a sampling frequency of 128 Hz give 2 seconds epoch.

There should be 256 points in the representation, which suffices for 128 amplitudes and 128 phases of the sines; that makes 128 points in the power spectrum, where we do not use the phase information. So, 128 points for a frequency range from 0 to 64 Hz give us 0.5-Hz distance between frequencies. If we would analyze 4 instead of 2 seconds, the resulting resolution would be 0.25 Hz.[3]

Generally, the longer sample (epoch) of an oscillation we have available for computation, the better we can determine its frequency. And, correspondingly, the shorter the time epoch, the less we know about frequency. Strictly speaking, time

3 Basically we can compute the products for as many frequencies as we like, but in general such oversampling will not improve the effective resolution, due to fluctuations and errors.

length is inversely proportional to the uncertainty of frequency determination, so the product of the time uncertainty (length of the epoch) and frequency uncertainty (distance between the points of the spectrum) is constant. This effect is known as the uncertainty principle in signal analysis. The corresponding theorem in physics is known as the Heisenberg principle—one of the counter-intuitive and "mysterious" properties of quantum mechanics. But if we look at Figure 3.11, the effect becomes quite obvious: what can we say about frequency, looking at just one or two points?

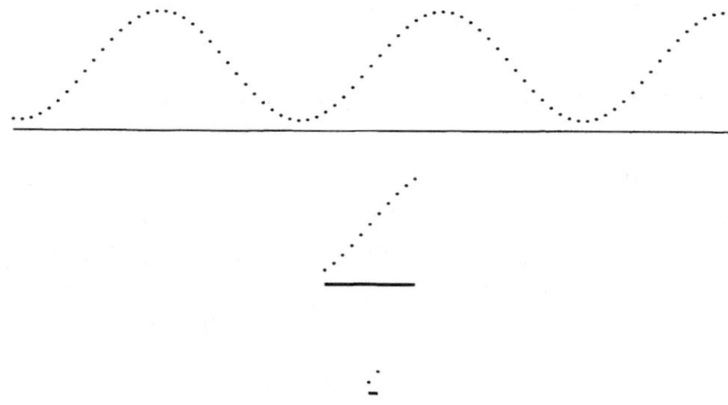

Figure 3.11 The uncertainty principle in signal analysis: the shorter the time epoch, the less we can say about the frequency. In the upper panel, the frequency of the oscillation can be determined from the samples with good accuracy, but we cannot assign it a well-defined point in time (the time spread is marked by the continuous solid line). If we improve the time determination (lower panels), shortening the epoch, then the very notion of frequency becomes disputable. In the limit of a perfect localization in time (one point), we cannot say anything about the frequency.

3.3 REAL-WORLD SPECTRA

Simulated signal from Section 3.1 can be explained using only two sine functions—this conclusion is presented in Figure 3.7. However, spectra computed for real-world signals are usually much more complicated and noisy due to the following reasons:

Noise is present in every real signal. It can result from the measurement process or analog/digital conversion. Also, a stochastic component is often an inherent part of the signal. Finally, the part of the signal that cannot be explained by the applied dictionary of functions or model is also treated as a noise. Noisy signal will give a noisy spectrum.

Transients are perfectly legal. We cannot expect all signals to be built from infinite oscillations: notes played on instruments start and end, conversations contain transient speech sounds—actually, it's their transient nature that makes these sounds interesting. However, spectra present only average properties of the signal and cannot account for the time variability. As an example, Figure 3.12 presents the power spectrum of a simulated, noiseless signal composed of two abruptly starting and ending sines and a single impulse.

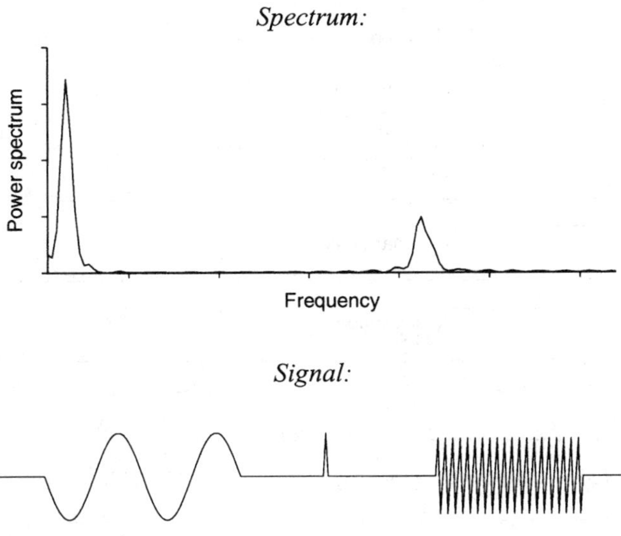

Figure 3.12 Signal containing transient oscillations and an isolated peak in the middle (lower plot) and its power spectrum (upper plot).

The spectrum indicates the presence of two oscillations of rather well-defined frequencies, but, obviously, we cannot deduce their time variations from the spectrum. And what happened to the impulse in the middle? As discussed in Section 3.2, we cannot assign a frequency to a one-point structure. Therefore, its energy is spread across the whole spectrum.

Nonsinusoidal oscillations, even if perfectly periodic, contain many harmonic frequencies needed to explain their nonsinusoidal shape. Figure 3.13 shows how many harmonics are needed to reasonably recover the shape of a rectangle.

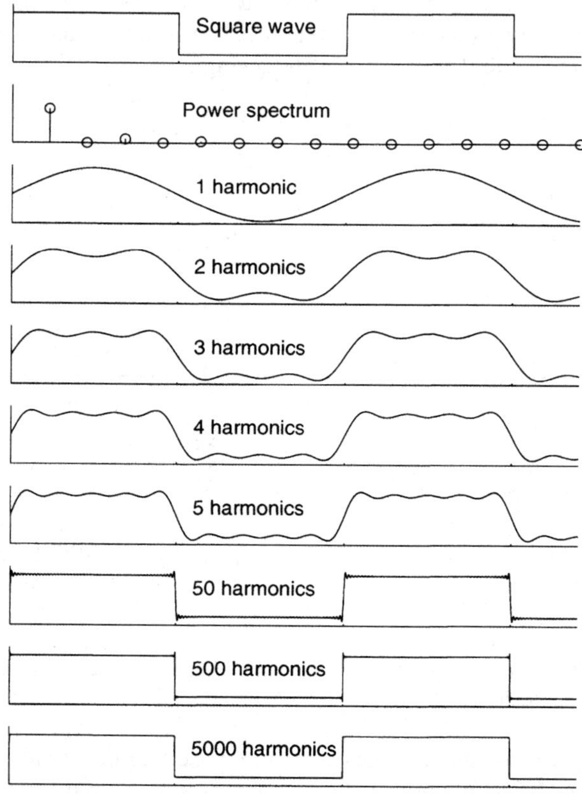

Figure 3.13 A square wave as a sum of sines: upper panel—an ideal continuous square wave. Second from the top—the first 15 points of the discrete power spectrum (i.e., relative energies of the sines from which the square wave can be reconstructed). Lower panels—reconstruction from the first 1–5, 50, 500, and 5000 sines (harmonic frequencies). Poor convergence at the edges of the square is called the Gibbs effect.

Chapter 4

Between Time and Frequency

This chapter introduces the classical time-frequency representations: short-time Fourier transform (STFT), spectrogram, and wavelet analysis, and discusses the issue of cross-terms in time-frequency estimates of signals energy density.

4.1 SPECTROGRAM

Let us get back to the issue of a time-varying spectral content of a signal. Using the methods developed in the previous chapter, we can start by computing the spectra on shorter subepochs of the signal. Such analysis is called short-time Fourier transform (STFT) or windowed Fourier transform (WFT). Plots of the magnitude of STFT are called spectrograms.

Instead of plotting a series of subsequent spectra, computed for the subsequent subepochs of the analyzed signal, we present the time evolution of frequencies in the *time-frequency plane*. The horizontal axis corresponds to time—just like when plotting a signal—and the vertical one is the frequency axis. Energy of the signal, occurring in given time and frequency ranges, can be marked by shades of gray.

Figure 4.1 presents the spectrogram of the signal, for which the spectrum was computed in Section 3.3. For comparison, the spectrum is plotted vertically on the left axis. Below the spectrogram, the original signal is plotted in the same time scale.

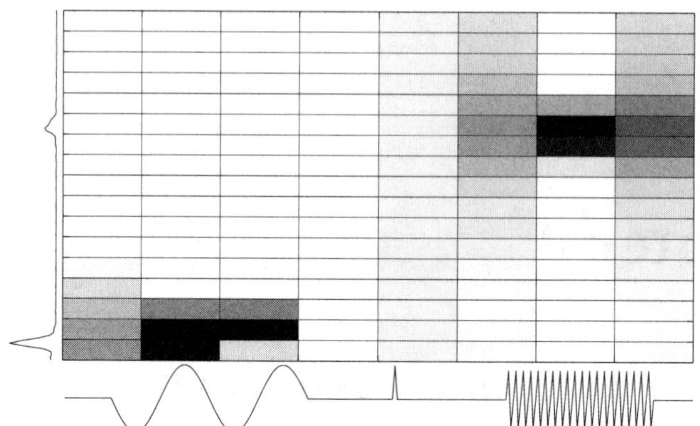

Figure 4.1 Spectrogram of the signal from Figure 3.12; the signal is plotted at the bottom. Vertical plot on the left represents its power spectrum. The horizontal axis for the spectrogram is the same as for the signal plotted below. The vertical axis denotes frequency, increasing upwards.

The central picture in Figure 4.1 is the time-frequency plane, divided into boxes, called "Heisenberg boxes," to stress the relation to the uncertainty principle in signal analysis, which does not allow us to estimate the energy density in arbitrarily small time-frequency regions (Section 3.2). The horizontal length of these boxes is chosen a priori and determines the time resolution of the representation. Their height, related to the frequency resolution, stems from the fixed tradeoff between the time length of the analyzed epoch and the frequency resolution of its spectrum.

This representation reflects some of the time-frequency characteristics of the signal: oscillation of lower frequency occurs in the first part of the signal, and the higher frequency is located closer to its end. But the price we pay for this information is a decreased accuracy of determination of the frequencies of these oscillations, comparing to the spectrum calculated for the whole epoch. For comparison, this spectrum is plotted vertically on the left axis.

The tradeoff between the time and frequency resolutions is regulated by the length of the analysis windows—in this case $\frac{1}{8}$ of the epoch. Is that length optimal? Unfortunately, there is no general answer to this question. Figure 4.2 presents spectrograms computed for the same signal using windows of different lengths, decreasing from the top. In the lower plots, corresponding to narrower windows, we start to notice an occurrence of a transient structure—the impulse located in the middle of the signal, which in the upper plots is completely diluted in relatively wide analysis windows. Energy of the impulse is spread across all the frequencies, which

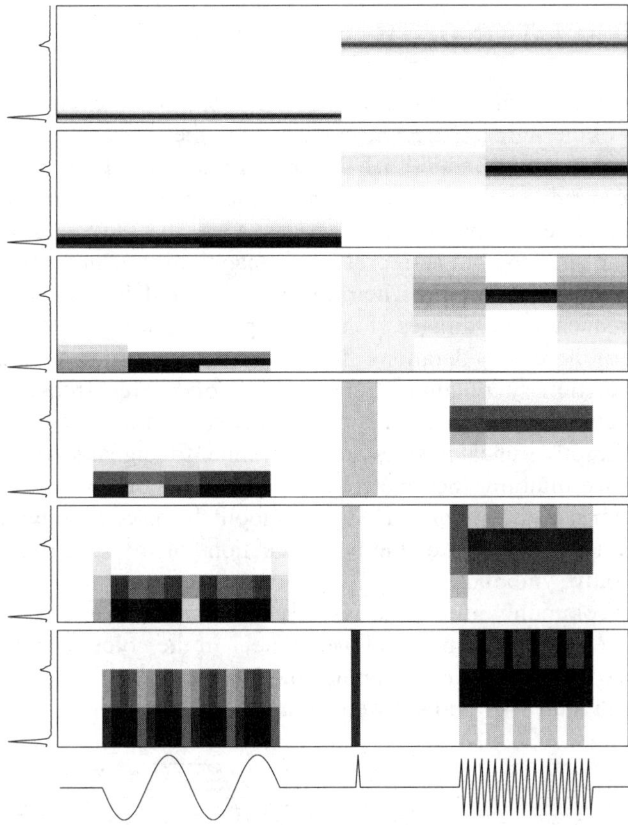

Figure 4.2 Spectrograms for the signal from Figure 3.12 (plotted at the bottom), computed for different window lengths: from a half-epoch window in the top plot to very narrow ones at the bottom. On the left axis, the spectrum is plotted vertically. Overlap of subsequent windows is set to zero.

relates to no frequency localization, stemming from the perfect localization in time (one point). But with increasing time resolution, the accuracy of determination of the frequencies of both oscillations degrades significantly.

4.2 INTERPRETATION OF THE SPECTROGRAM

In the previous section, the spectrogram was presented as a calculation of the spectra on subepochs of the signal. But let us come back to the meaning of "computing the spectra," as presented in Section 3.1. We recall that every point of the spectrum actually corresponds to the product of the signal with a sine of corresponding frequency (and optimal phase). Thus, we can view the shades of gray in every rectangle of the spectrogram as representing magnitudes of inner products of the signal with truncated sine waves. Their time positions and durations are determined by the time-frequency coordinates of the corresponding box.

In light of these considerations, the spectrogram can be viewed as explaining the signal in a dictionary containing truncated sines of different frequencies and time positions, but constant time widths. However, due to the issues discussed briefly in Section 3.3, abruptly truncated sines are not optimal for signal analysis, so in each time window we multiply the sine by a window function. We can use different window functions, as their goal is mostly to smooth the discontinuities at the edges. Therefore, the representation of the basic functions of the spectrogram, given in Figure 4.3, is only symbolic.

Another commonly used trick, visually enhancing the time resolution, relies on the use of overlapping time windows. Plate 1 in the color section presents, in panels (c) and (d), spectrograms computed in such a way. On the contrary, heuristic examples from Figures 4.1 and 4.2 were computed with no window overlap.

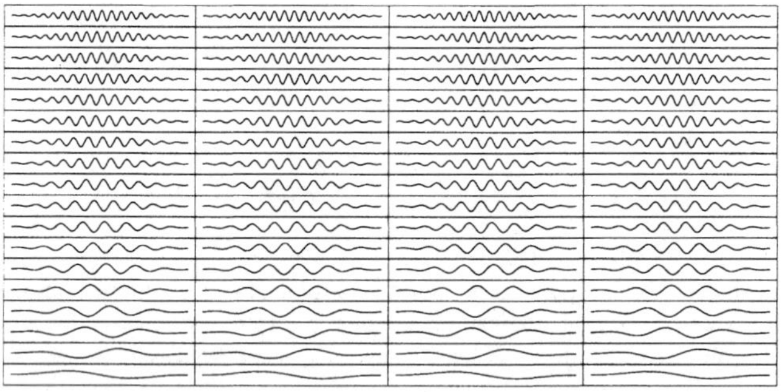

Figure 4.3 Shades of gray in Figures 4.1 and 4.2 represent the values of the product of the signal with sines of corresponding frequency and time span (and optimally fitted phase), modulated by a smoothing window. The above picture symbolically represents these sines, modulated by the Hamming window, in separate boxes. In practice we use overlapping windows—in this picture boxes would overlap in time.

4.3 WAVELETS

Windowed sines are not the only functions providing a reasonable localization in the time-frequency plane. We can construct time-frequency representations from an amazing variety of functions. In particular, one idea triggered the explosion of time-frequency signal analysis in the 1980s: *wavelets*.

This idea relates to a way of constructing the representation (or generating the dictionary), rather than to a particular function. For the wavelet, we can use any function that oscillates at least a bit and decays in ± infinity. Of course, different functions will yield different representations. Examples of wavelets are given in Figure 4.4.

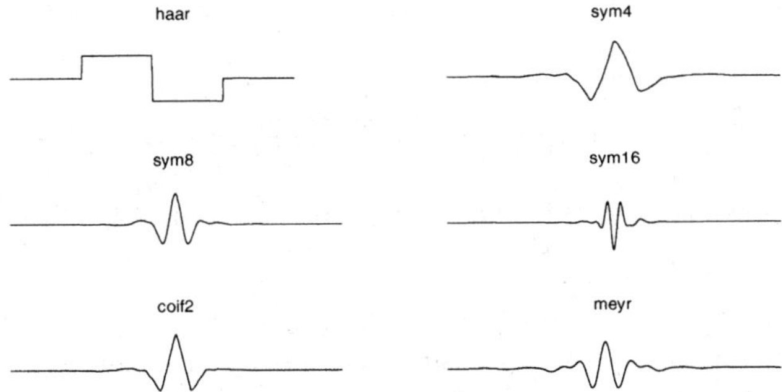

Figure 4.4 Some orthogonal wavelets. More examples and properties can be found in [1].

How can we explain different frequencies using these functions? Instead of modulating them explicitly with sines of varying frequencies, we stretch or dilate the one and fixed basic shape, as presented in Figure 4.5.

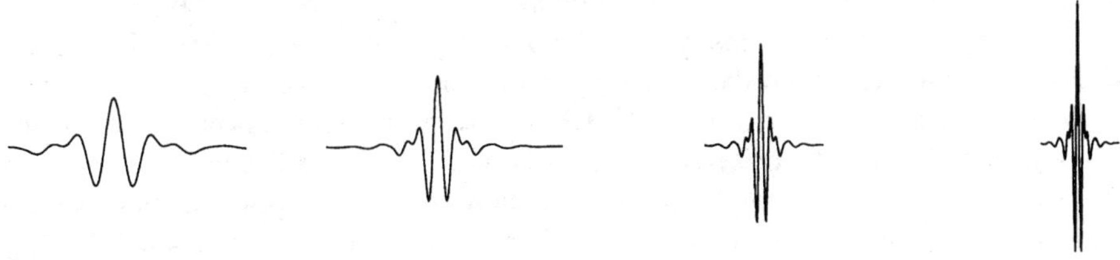

Figure 4.5 Scaling a wavelet. Each subsequent function is stretched twice, yielding a twice higher central frequency.

Stretching obviously brings the humps of the oscillations closer to each other, so a wavelet stretched twice will have a twice smaller distance between the humps, which corresponds to a twice higher central frequency. But this operation has one more important effect: a wavelet stretched twice effectively occupies a twice shorter time epoch and hence has a twice better time localization. And as we recall from Section 3.2, this also implies twice higher spread in frequency. Therefore, the Heisenberg boxes occupied by wavelets in the time-frequency plane, contrary to the uniform division offered by the spectrogram, will be distributed as in Figure 4.6.

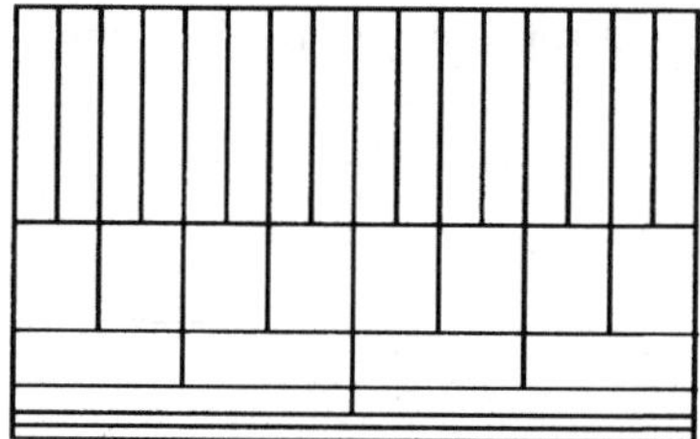

Figure 4.6 Symbolic division of the time-frequency plane in the wavelet transform. Corresponding picture for the spectrogram is given in Figure 4.3.

Owing to the "wavelet trick," which binds the frequency and time width, we achieve better time localization for structures of higher frequency. This is often desirable (e.g., in the detection of spikes). This effect is called the *zooming property* of wavelets. In Figure 4.7 we can observe this effect on the isolated pulse in the middle of the signal. However, we also notice poor determination of the higher frequency, especially compared to the spectrum plotted vertically on the left axis. In general, we say that wavelets offer a different tradeoff between time and frequency resolutions, where the time resolution improves—and frequency resolution degrades—for structures of higher frequency. It is an interesting alternative to the spectrogram, where we had to decide a priori the fixed width of the analysis window.

But is the wavelet transform really free of arbitrary choices? We already said that we can perform wavelet analysis using any of the variety of basic shapes (sometimes called "mother wavelets"). Obviously, representations computed using different wavelets will be different, as exemplified in Figure 4.8.

In particular, what triggered the explosion of wavelet applications in signal analysis was the mathematical discovery of a possibility of constructing orthogonal bases from translations and dilations of a single wavelet. This allowed for very efficient and fast algorithms for the calculation of the wavelet transform, which back in the 1980s was a significant factor. But the orthogonality is a still a desirable

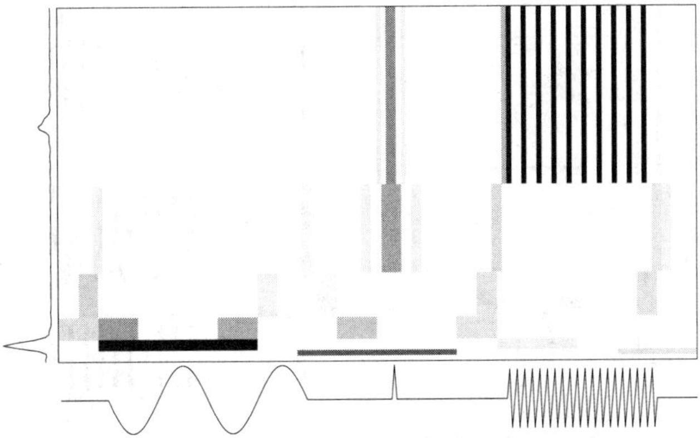

Figure 4.7 Wavelet transform of the signal from Figure 3.12 (plotted at the bottom). On the left axis, the spectrum is plotted vertically.

feature; all the wavelets from Figure 4.4, used for representation in Figure 4.8, generate orthogonal bases.

Finally, we must clarify that the representations presented in Figures 4.7 and 4.8 are called *discrete* wavelet transforms (DWT)—products are computed for as many wavelets as there are points in the signal.[1] To increase the resolution of the time-frequency picture, we can use tricks analogous to the sliding windows in the spectrogram. We can compute the products of the signal with *any* translation and dilation of the mother wavelet, yielding a smooth representation called continuous wavelet transform (CWT), as presented in Plate 1(b) in the color section.

4.4 WIGNER TRANSFORM AND CROSS-TERMS

When viewing results of the spectrogram (STFT) or wavelet transform (WT) in the time-frequency plane, like in Figures 4.2 and 4.8, we do not refer directly to the different dictionaries of the functions used in these transforms. Instead of products with these functions, we talk about overall estimates of time-frequency energy density, effectively treating the two-dimensional maps as the result of the analysis. This is most visible in the continuous wavelet transform and spectrograms computed with strongly overlapping windows, as in Plate 1(b)–(d). Such two-dimensional estimates

1 Contrary to the sines used in spectral estimates, for real-valued wavelets the phase information is fixed.

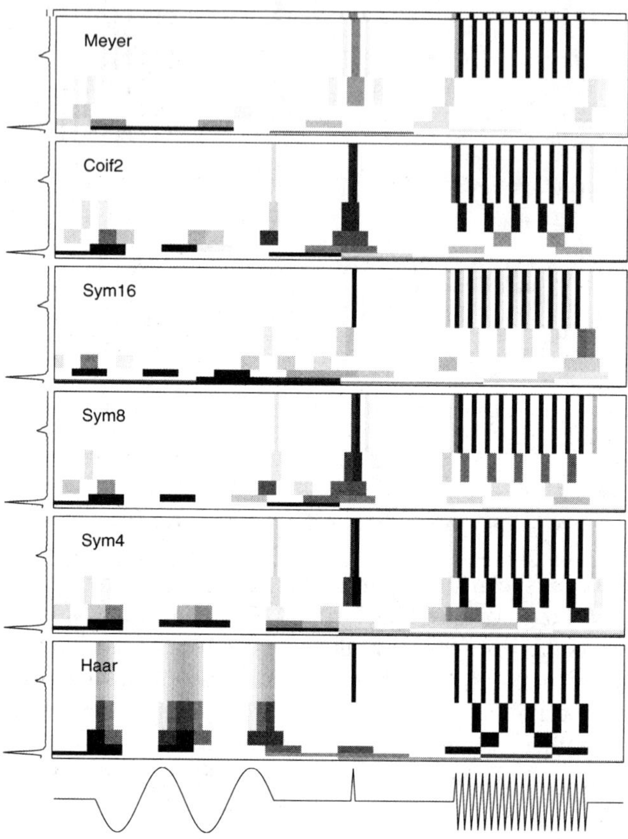

Figure 4.8 Wavelet transform of the signal from Figure 3.12 (plotted at the bottom), obtained with different wavelets from Figure 4.4. On the left axis, the spectrum is plotted vertically.

of the energy density of one-dimensional signals are mathematically *quadratic* transforms.

All these transforms share some general properties, like the tradeoff between the time and frequency resolutions. Another common problem—the presence of cross-terms—is best exemplified on the *Wigner transform*. Among the quadratic time-frequency representations, the Wigner transform occupies a central place, due to its mathematical elegance and some basic properties. However, in this case mathematical elegance does not translate directly into properties desirable in signal processing applications.

Figure 4.9 presents the Wigner transform of a signal similar to the one decomposed in previous sections—for clarity the impulse in the middle was removed, leaving only two sines with well-separated frequencies and time localizations. Comparing this picture to the previously calculated time-frequency estimates (Figures 4.2 and 4.8), we observe a very good localization of both the sines in time as well as frequency. Near the edges of the sines, the energy is less concentrated in frequency, but this is due to the discontinuities at the start and the end of the sines, which generate many harmonics (see, for example, Figure 3.13).

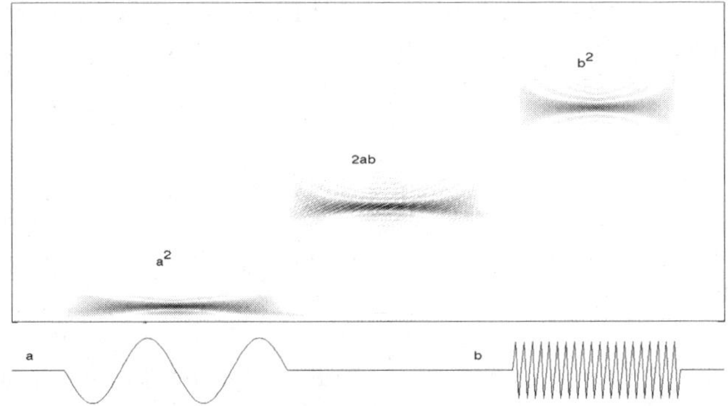

Figure 4.9 Wigner distribution (vertical-frequency, horizontal-time) of the signal simulated as two short sines (bottom). We observe the auto-terms a^2 and b^2 corresponding to the time and frequency spans of the sines, and cross-term $2ab$ at time coordinates where no activity occurs in the signal.

However, if we want to use the time-frequency picture as a tool for the inference about the content of an unknown signal, then the structure present in between these two is very frustrating. Actually, the Wigner transform indicates a high energy density in a time-frequency region, where obviously no activity is present! Unfortunately, this "false" structure—a cross-term—is not a calculation error, but an inherent feature of the Wigner transform. Due to such cross-terms, Wigner transform conserves some elegant marginal properties.

Cross-terms are present, to a different extent and in different forms, in *all* the quadratic time-frequency estimates of signal energy density. Wigner transform presents them in a raw form, convenient for understanding their properties. In particular, in the cross-term from Figure 4.9 we observe some repeating bars. Cross-terms, contrary to the auto-terms representing the actual signal structures, strongly oscillate. Therefore, smoothing the time-frequency representation can significantly decrease the contribution of cross-terms. But in a representation of an unknown signal, we cannot a priori smooth only the regions containing the cross-terms; therefore, the auto-terms will be also smoothed (smeared), resulting in a decreased time-frequency resolution.

The problem of cross-terms in signal processing has been recognized for years. Several mathematically advanced approaches have been developed to deal with it, for example by different ways of smoothing the Wigner transform (Section 13.3). Their detailed discussion is beyond the scope of this book (see, for example, [2, 3]). We just recall that to the discussed tradeoff between the time and frequency resolutions, we must add the tradeoff between the resolution and robustness/reliability (e.g., small contribution of cross-terms) present in the time-frequency estimates of signals energy density.

References

[1] I. Daubechies, *Ten Lectures on Wavelets*, Philadelphia, PA: Society for Industrial and Applied Mathematics, 1992.

[2] L. Cohen, *Time-Frequency Analysis*, Upper Saddle River, NJ: Prentice Hall, 1995.

[3] W. J. Williams, "Recent Advances in Time-Frequency Representations: Some Theoretical Foundations," in *Time Frequency and Wavelets in Biomedical Signal Processing*, M. Akay, (Ed.), IEEE Press Series in Biomedical Engineering, IEEE Press, Piscataway, NJ: 1997, pp. 3–44.

Chapter 5

Choosing the Representation

This chapter introduces adaptive time-frequency approximation of signals and the matching pursuit algorithm.

Each of the dictionaries discussed in previous chapters efficiently represents some kind of structures. Spectrogram (Section 4.1) describes oscillations with chosen time resolution, wavelets (Section 4.3) zoom nicely on singularities, and so on. In general, it is very hard to guess which dictionary would provide an optimal representation for a given signal. On the other hand, efficient and informative decomposition can be achieved only in a dictionary containing functions reflecting the structure of the analyzed signal. This rule, illustrated by numerous examples from previous sections, is hardly a surprise: *The limits of my language mean the limits of my world.*[1]

So, why don't we extend the limits—by constructing a big dictionary, rich enough to fit all the structures, possibly occurring in any signal of interest?

5.1 GABOR DICTIONARY

The most common approach to the construction of time-frequency dictionaries relies on Gabor functions, that is Gaussian envelopes modulated by sine oscillations. By multiplying these two functions, we can obtain a wide variety of shapes, depending on their parameters (Figures 5.1 and 5.2).

1 Ludwig Wittgenstein, *Tractatus Logico-Philosophicus*, thesis 5.6.

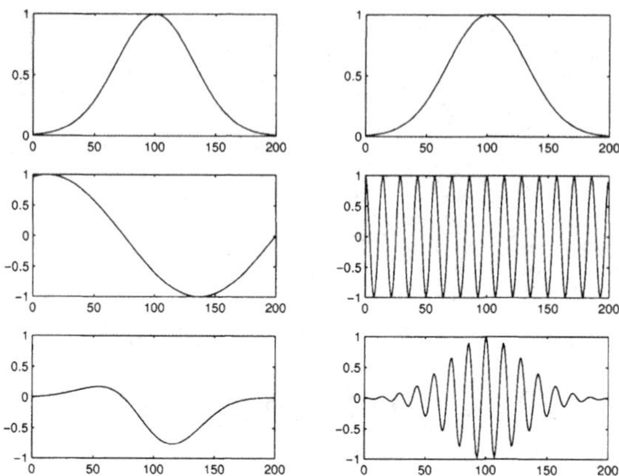

Figure 5.1 Gabor functions (bottom row) are constructed by multiplying Gaussian envelopes (upper row) with oscillations of different frequencies and phases (middle row).

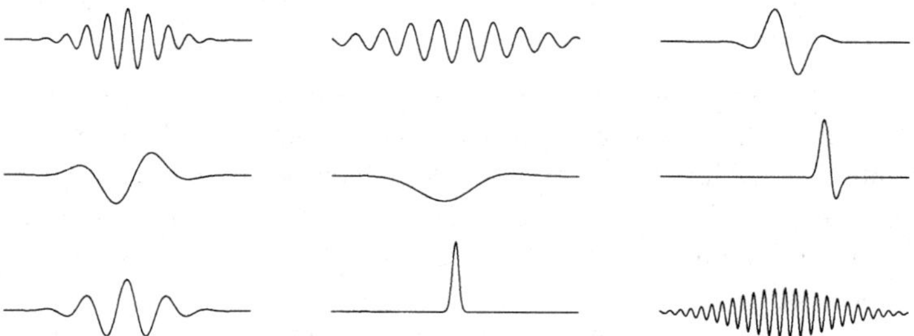

Figure 5.2 Examples of Gabor functions.

The advantage of this standardized approach is that all these different shapes, such as those presented in Figure 5.2 and many more,[2] can be described in terms of only four numbers per waveform: time width and position of the center of the Gaussian envelope, and frequency and phase of the modulating sine. Amplitudes are adjusted so that each function has equal (unit) energy, since the product of a waveform of unit energy with the signal will directly measure the contribution of that structure to the energy of the signal (product and energy were discussed in Section 2.1).

2 For example, pure sine waves and impulse functions can be treated as sines with very wide modulating Gauss and very narrow Gaussians, respectively.

Apart from the variety of shapes, there is a purely mathematical argument in favor of Gabor functions: they provide the best localization (lowest uncertainty, see Section 3.2) in the time-frequency plane [1]. However, this property is not crucial for understanding the procedure; the algorithm discussed in the next section can be used with any dense dictionary—that is, any dictionary containing at least enough functions to reproduce (efficiently or not) any signal.

5.2 ADAPTIVE APPROXIMATION

OK, we have a dictionary incorporating a variety of structures—how shall we use it? Following the classic approach described in the previous chapter for spectrogram and wavelets, we could try to use the products of all the functions from the dictionary with the signal. But in this case such representation would make no sense. If we use the whole dictionary of, say, millions of waveforms to describe 10 seconds of an EEG signal, we do not gain anything, either in terms of compression or understanding the signal structure. We must *choose* the representative waveforms. And if the choice will be adapted for each signal separately—unlike the a priori selections from Chapter 4—we may obtain a general, efficient, and adaptive procedure.

Matching pursuit is nothing but a procedure leading to such a choice. We will exemplify its operation on a signal composed of two Gabor functions and a little noise (Figure 5.3).

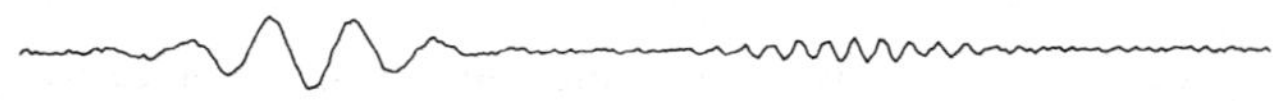

Figure 5.3 Signal constructed as a sum of two Gabor functions plus noise.

As the first candidate for the representation, we take the function, which, among all the functions from the dictionary, gives the largest product with the signal (Figure 5.4).

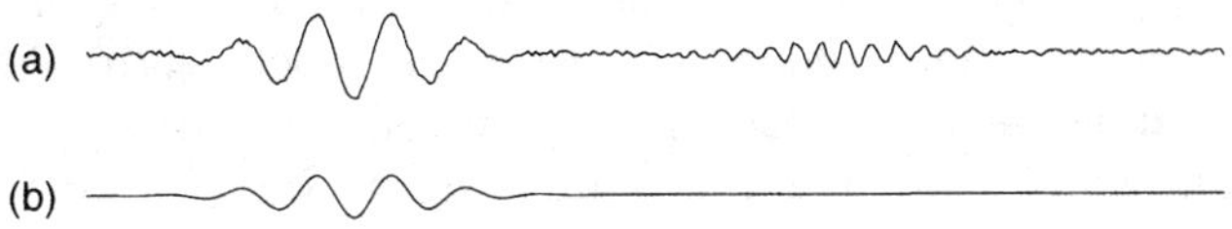

Figure 5.4 Function from the Gabor dictionary (b), giving the largest product with the signal (a).

However, a single function seldom explains exactly the whole signal. So, which function do we take as the second representative? The one giving the second largest product?

If the dictionary is rich, then it must contain many similar waveforms. One of them gives "the best fit" of the strongest structure. But the other, similar waveforms from the dictionary will most likely also fit the same structure—not "best," but still giving a large product. This product can be higher than the product of another, smaller structure, matched perfectly with a different waveform from the dictionary (Figure 5.5 (e)). Therefore, choosing *all* the waveforms that give a large product with the signal may result in a representation containing many similar waveforms, all approximating only the strongest structure of the signal—like (b), (c), and (d) from Figure 5.5—and completely omitting weaker structures, like (e).

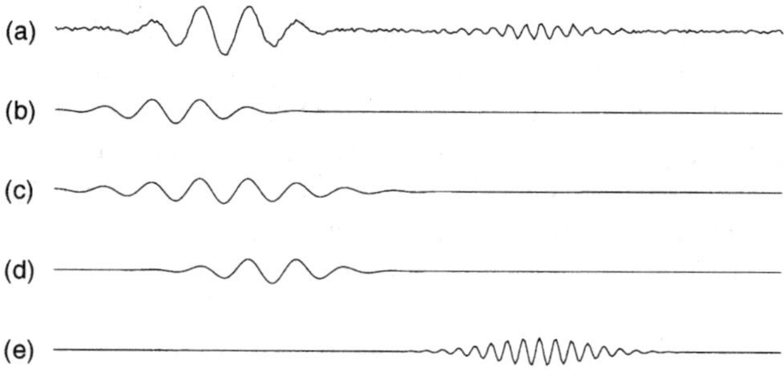

Figure 5.5 Similar functions from the dictionary (b–d) giving a large product with the signal (a). All these functions, more or less similar to the stronger structure, give larger products with the signal than the function exactly reflecting the weaker structure (e).

This is the price we pay for using a redundant dictionary. Smaller dictionaries, used in wavelet transform or STFT, are chosen so that their functions have little possible overlap—in the case of an orthogonal basis, the overlap is zero. If the dictionary were not so redundant, at most one of the functions (b), (c), and (d) in Figure 5.5 would be present. In such a case, we could use for the representation all the functions giving large products with the signal. But if the dictionary is so redundant, we must subtract the contribution of the first chosen function before fitting the next one.

5.3 MATCHING PURSUIT

Matching pursuit (MP) algorithm was first proposed in the context of signal analysis in 1993 by Mallat and Zhang in [2].[3] It is an iterative procedure, which can be described as follows:

1. Find (in the dictionary) the first function, that best fits the signal.
2. Substract its contribution from the signal.
3. Repeat these steps on the remaining residuals, until the representation of the signal in terms of chosen functions is satisfactory.

The first two iterations of this procedure, applied to the signal from Figure 5.3, are illustrated in Figure 5.6.

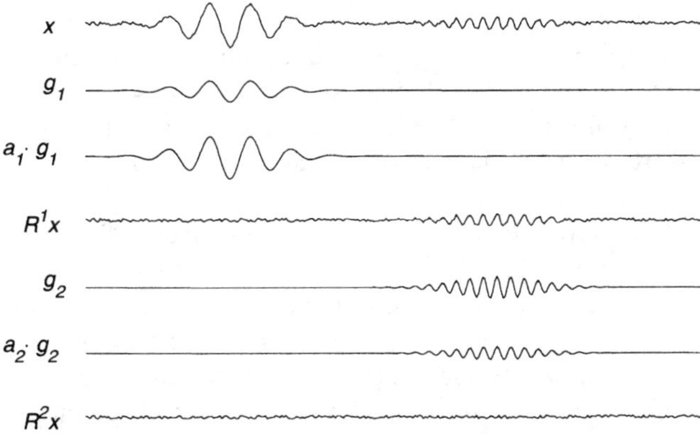

Figure 5.6 Matching pursuit algorithm. In the first step, we find the function g_1, which gives the largest product with the analyzed signal (x, upper trace). Then we adjust the amplitude of g_1 to the structure present in the signal and subtract it from the signal. The resulting (first) residual R^1x does not contain the contribution explained by the first fitted function. Therefore, the next function (g_2), found in the dictionary as giving the largest product with the residual, will fit the next structure present in the signal. If these two functions (g_1 and g_2) give a satisfactory representation of the signal x (e.g., explains the required percentage of energy), we can stop the procedure at this point and leave R^2x as the unexplained residual.

3 A similar approach to signals was proposed in [3]. The general idea was known previously from statistics as a regression pursuit.

As a result, we obtain an approximation of the signal x in terms of the functions g_1 and g_2 and their amplitudes a_1 and a_2, plus the unexplained residual:

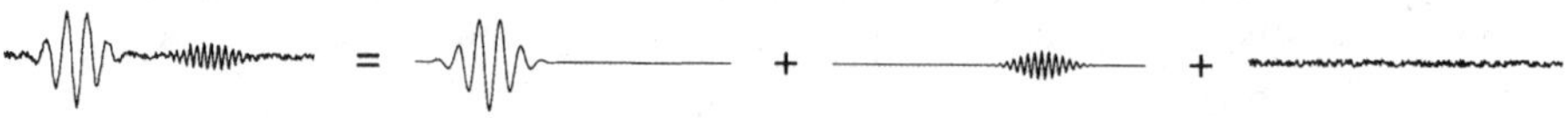

= + +

or

$$x = a_1 \cdot g_1 + a_2 \cdot g_2 + R^2 x \ ,$$

where $R^2 x$ denotes the residual of signal x left after the second iteration.

5.4 TIME-FREQUENCY ENERGY DENSITY

So, we have a nice and compact description of the signal in terms of a sum of known functions. What about the picture of its time-frequency energy density?

First, let us recall the meaning of such a picture. As an image, it naturally has two dimensions. The horizontal dimension corresponds to time, and its extent reflects the length of the analyzed epoch. Vertical dimension represents frequency and may extend from zero to the half of the sampling frequency (i.e., the Nyquist frequency).[4]

Graphically we represent the energy density as shades of gray, color scale, or height in 3-D plots. If the signal has a high-energy activity of a given frequency in a given time epoch, we expect the corresponding area of the picture to exhibit high values of energy density. In the previous chapters we used a fixed set of functions (e.g., sines or wavelets), so we could a priori divide the time-frequency plane into boxes corresponding to these functions. Examples of such pictures are given in Figures 4.1 and 4.2 (spectrograms) and 4.7 and 4.8 (orthogonal wavelet transforms).

Using the matching pursuit expansion, we do not know a priori which functions will be chosen for the representation. The decomposition is adaptive, so we cannot draw a prior division of the time-frequency plane like in Figures 4.3 or 4.6. But for each of the functions, chosen for the representation of the signal, we can compute the corresponding time-frequency distribution of energy density, by means of the Wigner transform (Section 4.4). For the Gabor functions from the dictionary discussed in Section 5.1, we obtain blobs in the time-frequency plane extending in time approximately in the regions of the represented structures.[5] Their frequency

4 We recall from Section 1.2 that Nyquist frequency is the maximum frequency which can be reliably detected in a digital signal.

5 This ellipsoidal blob is actually a 2-D Gauss function.

extent is determined by the uncertainty principle (Section 3.2), which states that the shorter the structure is in time, the wider is its frequency content. An impulse can be considered an extremely short structure, so it will be represented as a vertical line. Infinite sine will be infinitely narrow in frequency, so it will make a horizontal line. By adding energy densities for all the functions from the decomposition, we obtain representations like in Figure 5.7.

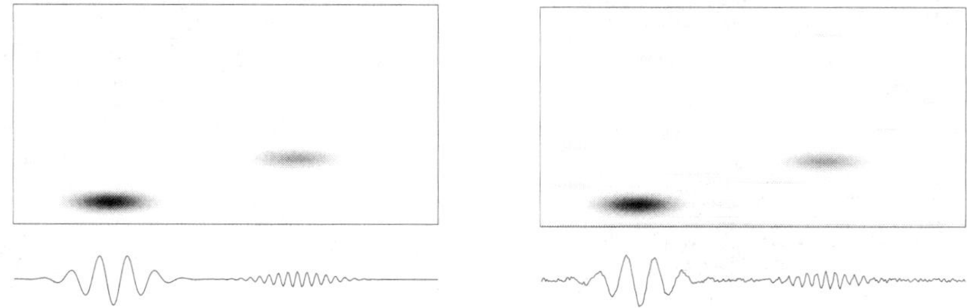

Figure 5.7 Left: sum of the first two functions (g_1 and g_2 from Figure 5.6) and its time-frequency energy density. Right: time-frequency representation of the signal from Figure 5.3, including noise. Apart from the same two structures representing the major components of the signal, we observe a lot of weaker blobs distributed uniformly across the time-frequency plane, representing the white noise added in simulation to the two structures. Vertical axis corresponds to frequency, increasing upwards.

But what do we actually gain from this approach, compared to the direct calculation of the Wigner transform of the signal, as in Section 4.4? From the matching pursuit decomposition, we know (or assume) that the signal is a sum $g_1 + g_2$. Using this information, we do not have to take the Wigner transform of the whole sum (i.e., the whole signal), which would give $g_1^2 + g_2^2 + 2g_1g_2$, but instead we take only $g_1^2 + g_2^2$, that is the sum of energy densities of the components, not including cross-terms. The problem of cross-terms is exemplified in Figure 4.9.

Figure 5.8 presents decompositions of a bit more complex signal, constructed from a continuous sine wave, one-point impulse (Dirac's delta), and three Gabor functions. Panel (b) gives time-frequency energy distribution obtained for this signal from MP decomposition. In the left, three-dimensional plots, energy is proportional to the height. In the right two-dimensional maps, energy is coded in shades of gray. Panels (c) and (d) present decompositions of the same signal with addition of a white noise of energy twice and four times the signal's energy. We observe basically retained representation of the major signal structures (slightly disturbed in the presence of the stronger noise) and a uniform distribution of the noise-related, weaker structures.

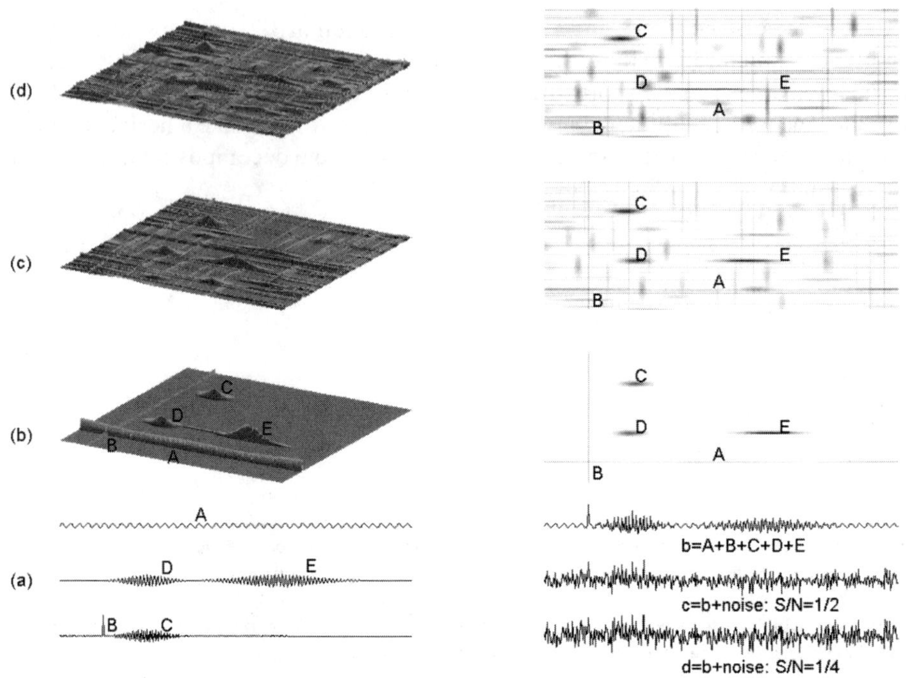

Figure 5.8 (a): Left—components of the simulated signal: sine A, Dirac's delta B, and Gabor functions C, D, and E. Right—signals, labelled b, c, and d, constructed as sum of structures A–E and white noise, and decomposed in corresponding panels (b), (c), and (d). (b): Time-frequency energy density obtained for sum of structures *A–E*; in 3-D representation on the left, energy is proportional to the height, while in the right panel it is proportional to the shades of gray. Panels (c) and (d): decompositions of signals with linear addition of noise, S/N = 1/2 (−3 dB) in (c) and −6 dB in (d). The same realization of white noise was used in both cases. (Reprinted from [4] with permission. © 2001 by PTBUN and IBD.)

References

[1] S. Mallat, *A Wavelet Tour of Signal Processing*, 2nd ed., New York: Academic Press, 1999.

[2] S. Mallat and Z. Zhang, "Matching Pursuit with Time-Frequency Dictionaries," *IEEE Transactions on Signal Processing*, vol. 41, December 1993, pp. 3397–3415.

[3] S. Qian and D. Chen, "Signal Representation Using Adaptive Normalized Gaussian Functions," *Signal Processing*, vol. 36, March 1994, pp. 1–11.

[4] K. J. Blinowska and P. J. Durka, "Unbiased High Resolution Method of EEG Analysis in Time-Frequency Space," *Acta Neurobiologiae Experimentalis*, vol. 61, 2001, pp. 157–174.

Chapter 6

Advantages of Adaptive Approximations

This chapter briefly summarizes those features of the matching pursuit that are unique among the currently available signal processing methods, as well as the advantages they offer in the analysis of biomedical signals.

6.1 EXPLICIT PARAMETERIZATION OF TRANSIENTS

Matching pursuit[1] (MP) breaks down the analyzed signal into a weighted sum of known functions (i.e., waveforms of well-defined time and frequency centers, width, amplitude, and phase). These functions represent the structures—oscillations and transients—present in the signal. It may sound obvious after reading the last two sections, so let us see why is it so special and how can we explore this feature.

None of the previously applied signal processing methods provides direct and explicit parameterization of both transient and oscillatory phenomena. For example, Fourier transform, described in Chapter 3,[2] gives average characteristics of the whole analyzed epoch: there is no way to tell whether oscillations, reflected by a

1 Matching pursuit is an iterative algorithm finding a suboptimal solution to the problem of an optimal representation of a signal in redundant dictionary (Section 13.4). It is the most popular and efficient solution, currently the only one which can be recommended for practical applications. Other possible solutions or modifications of MP are mentioned in Sections 13.6 and 13.11. Mathematical formalism of MP and related technical issues are introduced in Section 13.5.

2 As well as other methods of estimating spectra, such as those based upon the autoregressive (AR) model.

peak in the spectrum, occur across the whole epoch or only its part. Classical time-frequency methods, like spectrogram, wavelets, or Wigner transform, mentioned in Chapter 4, estimate the time evolution of the spectrum, providing distributions of signal energy in the time-frequency plane. These distributions are two-dimensional maps, like those presented in Plate 1 in the color section, Figures 4.2, 4.8, 4.9, and the upper panel of Figure 6.1. We can try to deduce from such maps the appearance of certain structures in the signal, but this deduction is only indirect, as it requires some kind of post-processing or analysis—usually visual—of these maps.[3] Finally, there is a variety of detection algorithms, usually based upon template matching techniques, that returns only signal correlation with given pattern.

Let us recall the form of results provided by adaptive time-frequency approximations. The actual output of matching pursuit is given in terms of numbers—parameters of the functions, fitted to the signal. Figure 6.1 presents this output as

1. Parameters of Gabor functions, listed explicitly in the shaded boxes;
2. Time courses of the corresponding Gabor functions (middle, gray plots);
3. Two-dimensional blobs representing concentrations of energy density in the time-frequency plane, corresponding to functions from the MP expansion.

Time-frequency maps of energy are explored in Chapter 10; reconstructions are indirectly used in Sections 8.6 and 8.7. However, here we treat these maps and reconstructions only as a sometimes convenient visualization of the primary output of the MP algorithm—parameters of chosen functions. These parameters provide an exact and complete description of the signal structures, in terms of their time occurrence (center and width, or start and end) *and* frequency center *and* amplitude *and* phase. These numbers can be used *directly* to identify those functions from the MP expansion that correspond to the signal's structures of interest. Identification can be accomplished via one of the two major approaches—or their mix/iteration:

1. Filters for selecting relevant structures, operating on the parameters of fitted functions (e.g., ranges of time widths, frequencies, and amplitudes), can be constructed a priori, based upon existing definitions of the waveforms (e.g. sleep spindles or slow waves).

3 As illustrated in the mentioned figures, such an interpretation can be prone to a significant error, depending on the relation between the chosen method/parameters and the actual content of the signal.

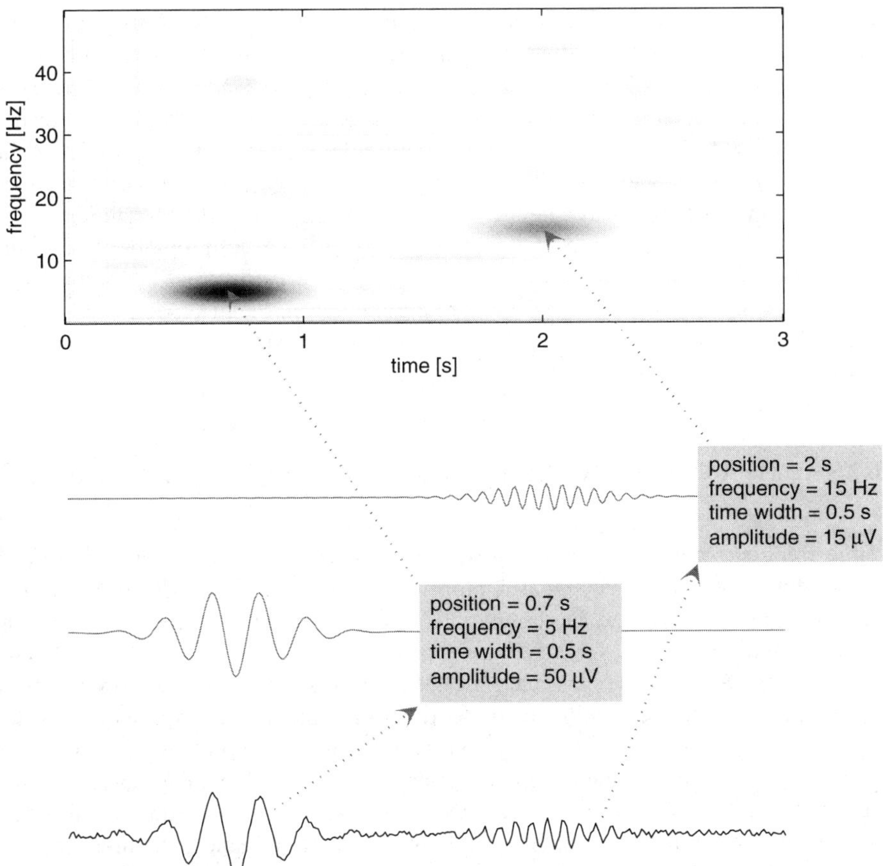

Figure 6.1 MP decomposition of a simulated signal (lower plot, black) from Figures 5.6 and 5.7, containing two Gabor functions and a little noise. Shaded boxes present parameters of the Gabor functions, fitted to the signal in the first two MP iterations. These numbers can be used either to reproduce the time courses of these functions, plotted in gray as middle traces, or the time-frequency distribution of signal's energy density, presented in the upper panel (this representation was computed from a larger number of iterations). Blobs corresponding to the first two iterations are indicated by arrows; remaining structures in the time-frequency plane represent the noise.

2. Time-frequency parameters, defining the relevant waveforms, can be deduced a posteriori—by investigating MP representations of signal epochs containing the structures of interest.

In both these cases, a posteriori agreement with the relevant criterion (visual or other) can be used to adjust the parameters. For example, as mentioned in Section 8.3, MP-based detection of delta waves was first approached directly—that is, using the classical parameters defined in the manuals, which included a fixed 75-μV threshold for the minimum amplitude. However, a comparison of the preliminary results with visual detection performed by human experts revealed that experienced electroencephalographers instinctively lower the threshold of slow wave's amplitude in the case of a generally lower EEG amplitude observed in the whole recording. This compensation for intersubject variability was later introduced in the detection algorithm, using linear relation between the mean amplitude of the whole EEG recording and the minimum amplitude of a slow wave.

6.2 AUTOMATIC NEGOTIATION OF TIME-FREQUENCY TRADEOFF

Time-frequency distribution of energy density provides important information about the content of an unknown signal. Unfortunately, there are many different ways in which we can compute this representation—thus, we should speak about computing given estimate.

Computation of the classical time-frequency estimates is based upon a prior choice of parameter, regulating the tradeoff between the time and frequency resolutions. In the spectrogram (short-time Fourier transform), this is the width of the time window; for the wavelet transform, this tradeoff is regulated by the properties of the chosen wavelet—as discussed in Sections 4.1 and 4.3. Figures 4.2 and 4.8 illustrate differences between time-frequency estimates computed using the same methods (spectrogram with nonoverlapping windows and orthogonal wavelet transforms), but with different settings of the corresponding parameters, regulating the time-frequency tradeoff.

Plate 1 further exemplifies this ambiguity by presenting several estimates, computed for the same signal using different methods. The signal is plotted at the bottom right in black, its components at the bottom left in red. Panel (b) presents continuous wavelet transform; panels (c) and (d) give smooth spectrograms, obtained by sliding windows with large overlap. These estimates, as discussed previously, depend heavily on the prior choice of wavelet or window length. We can also observe the inherent difference between these two types of transforms. Spectrogram maintains constant time-frequency resolution, resulting from the prior setting of the window length. Wavelet transform gives perfect time localization of the impulse present in the middle of the signal, clearly marked in high frequencies. This comes at a cost of degrading the frequency resolution with increasing frequency.

Panel (e) of Plate 1 presents a Wigner transform of the same signal. Compared to Figure 4.9, the signal contains more structures, which results in heavy cross-term contamination of the Wigner estimate of energy density. Cross-terms make this representation useless for a direct inference about the content of an unknown signal. However, we also observe that some auto-terms, like the inclined line running from the lower left to the upper right corner, provide an almost perfect representation[4] of the structures (in this case, a chirp) present in the signal.

As mentioned in Sections 4.4 and 13.3, we can reduce the cross-terms in a Wigner distribution by smoothing the time-frequency representation. The choice of a smoothing kernel relates to the settings of the time-frequency resolution present in other representations. Panel (f) presents the results of such smoothing. We observe a slightly diluted width of the line representing the chirp, some little cross-terms here and there, but overall, the picture represents very well all the structures present in the signal. Contrary to representations from (b)–(e), we can easily guess the presence of the changing frequency (chirp), four time-limited structures of different frequencies (Gabor functions), and, a bit less obvious, sine and impulse.[5] Unfortunately, there is a catch: the smoothing kernel used to compute this representation was found and adjusted by a trial-and-error procedure aimed at best representing the *known* structure of the simulated signal. If we use the same kernel for representation of a different signal, the chances that mostly auto-terms will be preserved and cross-terms will be minimized are very little.

Finally, panel (g) gives the time-frequency estimate computed from MP decomposition. We observe very good representation of the four Gabor functions, and, less pronounced but still clear, traces of the sine and impulse. However, the chirp, which was so clearly visible in the smoothed Wigner transform, now appears as a series of separate blobs. This is due to the fact that in the dictionary used for MP decomposition, there are only structures of constant frequency. This exemplifies again that to properly interpret a time-frequency picture of a signal's energy density, we need an extra information about how was it estimated. Nevertheless, the MP estimate stands out in several points. First of all, we may wonder why there is only one MP estimate presented. Contrary to spectrograms computed using different

4 Theoretical representation of a linear chirp (that is, sine with linearly increasing frequency) is a slanted line, infinite sine of constant frequency would be a horizontal line, and an ideal impulse—a vertical line.

5 In this signal, sine and impulse carry relatively little energy (i.e., they are weak compared to the other structures). Spotting their presence may require some intuition on the usual appearance of cross-terms.

windows, all the MP decompositions of the same signal in the Gabor dictionary will look at least very similar (with differences only due to the implementation details). In all the estimates but the matching pursuit, time-frequency resolution has to be decided a priori—by choosing the analyzing window of the spectrogram, properties of the wavelet, smoothing kernel of the Wigner transform, and so forth. On the contrary, MP adapts the resolution to each structure separately, to provide its optimal representation (in terms of the applied dictionary)—no prior setting of this tradeoff is required by the procedure.

As described in Sections 5.4 and 13.10, due to the explicit parameterization of signal structures, we can exclude the cross-terms from the time-frequency picture. Although this exclusion is perfect only when the signal is perfectly modelled by the expansion, even in cases when the parameterization is far from ideal, like representation of the chirp by a series of Gabor functions, the overall picture is still robust. It does not display a high energy density in the area where no activity occurs in the signal.

Getting back to the description of the MP algorithm in Section 5.3, we can understand these features as stemming from an *automatic* choice of the proper width of the Gabor function, which regulates the time-frequency tradeoff in the Gabor dictionary, in each step (iteration). This choice is based upon a simple criterion, maximizing the amount of energy explained in each step.

6.3 FREEDOM FROM ARBITRARY SETTINGS

Using most of the classical methods of signal analysis, we are responsible for a proper choice of parameters, which may bias the results. These parameters, related to the time-frequency resolution, have to be adjusted to the properties of a particular signal, depending also on the scope of its analysis. Interpretation of results requires taking into account the influence of these settings, sometimes by comparing different estimates computed for the same signal. On the contrary, issues related to a correct MP decomposition and its interpretation can be treated to a large extent separately.

As discussed in previous sections, MP adapts the tradeoff between time and frequency resolutions to the local content of the signal, in this respect eliminating the need for prior settings. The only parameters affecting the decomposition—the density/structure of the applied dictionary and the number of iterations—are discussed in Chapter 7. However, both these parameters obey the general rule "the larger, the better," and so reflect rather a tradeoff between the accuracy and the computational cost of the procedure. Therefore, we can simply talk about a "good," or "properly computed," MP decomposition. On the contrary, in the case of the other estimates, we have to take into account the influence of prior choices related to the time-frequency tradeoff and the fit between these parameters and the properties of the analyzed signal.

6.4 A UNIFIED FRAMEWORK

Freedom from arbitrary settings, discussed in the previous section, greatly simplifies the comparison of results from different studies, based upon properly computed MP decompositions, since we do not have to take into account possibly different settings of the time-frequency resolutions. In this section we would like to highlight the fact that the same MP decomposition can be applied in a variety of ways in different signal processing contexts. In all the tasks presented in this book, we can use the same, general MP decomposition, computed only once for a given signal. Based upon this decomposition, we compute different measures, related to the relevant features of the signal, as a specific postprocessing of this relatively universal parameterization. This facilitates drawing results from different measures applied to similar phenomena, which previously were usually quantified in different contexts using significantly different methods.

Let us take, for example, sleep spindles. These typical EEG structures were first described and parameterized in the context of visual EEG analysis. Subsequently, detection of their occurrences was attempted using a variety of signal processing algorithms, aimed at agreement with detection of human experts. Of course different algorithms are giving different results in comparison to different groups of experts. At the same time, spectral integrals—computed usually in a priori selected bands—were used as an overall measure of the spindling activity in a given EEG epoch. In special cases, mixtures of these approaches were used. For example, spectral powers of visually selected epochs containing sleep spindles were used for spatial localization of their generators—this case is discussed in Section 12.4.

This situation raises a fundamental question whether—or rather to what extent—in all these different approaches we are indeed dealing with the same phenomena. This issue is automatically solved within the MP-based framework, presented in this book. MP-based detection of relevant structures can be first investigated and fine-tuned using the available definitions and agreement with visual detection or any other available criteria—for sleep spindles we can, for example, implement directly their definitions from the electroencephalographers' manuals (Section 8.2). Once we are satisfied with the results, we can use exactly the same procedure of parameterization of relevant structures to compute (a) detection-related measures related to their occurrences, (b) power carried by these structures, or (c) completely new measures. In case of sleep spindles, the number of their occurrences per minute (relevant for staging) is presented in Figure 8.5. As exemplified in the same figure, using MP parameterization we can also compute power carried by *the same structures* in subsequent sleep epochs. The same power estimate can be used quantitatively in pharmaco EEG, bringing not only elegance and confidence of dealing with the relevant phenomena, but also significant improvement of sensitivity (Section 11.2). Similar improvement can be achieved in spatial localization by combining multichannel MP parameterization of sleep spindles with EEG inverse solutions (Section 12.4).

From the same decomposition we can also compute measures used in visual EEG analysis, like the percentage of an epoch occupied by given structures (Figure 8.7), which were unavailable from the previously applied signal processing methods, or completely new measures of signal complexity, like the Gabor Atom Density introduced in epilepsy research (Section 9.4). Finally, we can use exactly the same MP parameterization for computing a robust estimate of time-frequency energy density, as discussed in the previous two sections and further explored in Chapter 10.

Of course this is an optimistic picture, and not all the problems and structures present in biomedical signals must yield such promising results as the examples described in this book. But it seems that in many cases it's at least worth a try.

Chapter 7

Caveats and Practical Issues

This chapter discusses possible errors one can make in MP decomposition—by using too small a dictionary or too few waveforms in the expansion. A third error can result from misinterpretation of results involving a possible statistical bias, but this one comes into play only when processing large amounts of data.

7.1 DICTIONARY DENSITY

Up to now we viewed the MP algorithm as simply "choosing in each step the best Gabor function." In theory this can indeed be any Gabor, but in practice we must limit the dictionary D of candidate functions to some finite set. Due to the simple strategy taken by the MP algorithm, which relies on computing inner products of the signal[1] with all the candidate functions and choosing the one that gives the largest value, the size of this set heavily influences the computational cost of the procedure. Some tricks that can decrease the computational complexity of this procedure are described in Chapter 14; for example, we do not have to include in the dictionary explicitly Gabor functions with different phases (Section 14.1).

Obviously, for analysis of a longer epoch of a signal, we need a dictionary containing more candidate functions—more possible translations in time and widths can be reasonably fitted to a longer signal. Also frequency resolution increases with the length of the epoch, as mentioned in Section 3.2, so for a longer signal we can

1 Or, in later iterations than the first, with the residuum.

reasonably also sample the frequency parameters with finer resolution. Because of that, we should talk about a density rather than the size of a dictionary. This density is measured in the time-frequency-scale space, so it need not be linearly related to the length of the signal (see Section 13.8). In any case, the basic facts related to the size of the dictionary in practical implementations of MP are simple:

Good news: Using too big a dictionary in MP decomposition will not degrade the quality of resulting representation.

Bad news: There is no general recipe for a "large enough" dictionary. Too small a dictionary may degrade the quality of representation. Increasing the size of the dictionary increases the computational burden of the MP procedure.

Obviously, this is not a tradeoff between conflicting but desirable properties of the representation, like in case of the time-frequency tradeoff, but rather a price/performance kind of choice.

In a typical signal processing applications, optimal size of the MP dictionary is usually addressed within the rate distortion framework, searching for a minimum rate (amount of information) that should be communicated (or stored) to reproduce the input signal with given distortion. As a distortion we can take (the energy of) the difference between the MP expansion and the original signal. But the minimum amount of information (that is, bits) needed to store the results of MP decomposition depends not only on the number of waveforms included in the expansion, but also on the number of waveforms present in the applied dictionary. For example, if we have a relatively small dictionary, we can simply number all the functions and store only the indices of selected waveforms and their weights. On the other hand, with a small dictionary, we usually need more waveforms to explain the given percentage of a signal's energy (i.e., achieve the same distortion). These issues are crucial in applications aiming at maximum compression with minimum loss of information, like video coding (see [1–3]).

However, in the analysis of biomedical signals, we do not want to risk missing an important feature (e.g., an epileptic spike) in exchange for decreasing memory usage. Therefore we prefer to use rich repertoires of functions—large dictionaries. Fortunately, the price of computational resources drops very fast due to the progress in computer hardware. Therefore, recent software packages implementing the MP decomposition should offer reasonable defaults in terms of "large enough" dictionary sizes, calculated automatically for the size of the decomposed signal. But it is still one of the parameters that we may like to control and adjust for particular tasks.

7.2 NUMBER OF WAVEFORMS IN THE EXPANSION

Let us recall that MP is an iterative algorithm, and that the number of iterations performed before stopping the procedure equals the number of waveforms in the resulting signal expansion.

Bad news: There are several different criteria for stopping the MP algorithm.

Good news: Functions in MP expansions are ordered by energy, and subsequent iterations do not influence the previous steps.[2]

The effect of using a different number of waveforms for computing a time-frequency estimate for the same signal is illustrated in Figure 7.1.

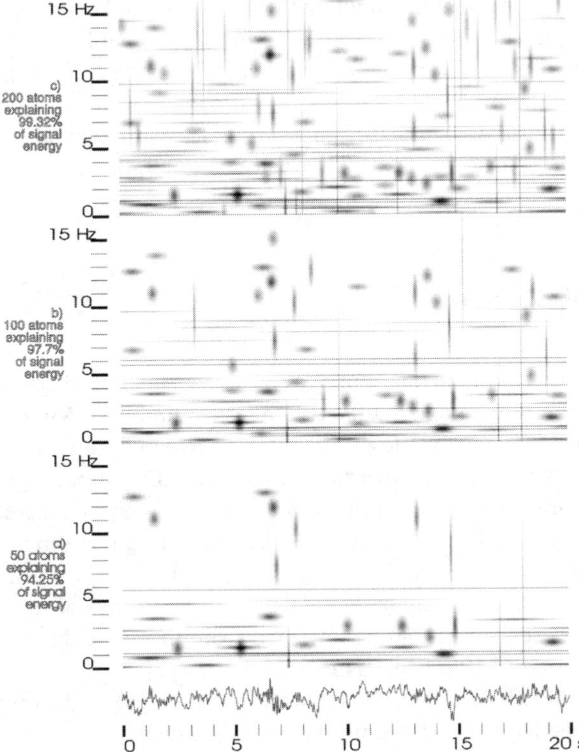

Figure 7.1 Time-frequency maps of energy, computed for the same signal with different numbers of functions in MP expansions.

2 This may not be the case for some of the modifications of MP discussed in Section 13.6.

The most important feature of the MP decomposition (in relation to the number of waveforms), visible in Figure 7.1, is that the strongest signal structures are represented by exactly the same time-frequency blobs in all the decompositions, regardless of the number of waveforms used in the expansion. It is a result of the greedy and short-sighted strategy of choice employed in the MP algorithm discussed in Section 13.11. However, in the context of stability related to the number of iterations, this feature is a big advantage. Since the subsequent iterations do not influence the previous ones, the first M functions—in decompositions of the same signal using the same dictionary—will always be the same. In other words, we do not have to use all the functions. As discussed in Section 13.7, after explaining the part of the signal coherent with the dictionary, further iterations may carry no information, as representing functions fitted to noise. But even if we stop the procedure later, which corresponds to a larger than reasonable number of functions in the expansion, this will in no way influence or degrade the information carried by the functions fitted in lower iterations.

Stopping criteria are discussed in Section 13.7, and a practical example of their relevance for a particular task is given in Section 9.4.

7.3 STATISTICAL BIAS

Statistical bias is discussed in detail in Section 13.9. This issue should be taken into account when pooling together results from a large number of MP decompositions. An example of its effect is visible in Figure 7.2, presenting a frequency histogram of sleep spindles detected in an overnight EEG recording. Looking at the left histogram, we may draw a conclusion of the prevalence of certain discrete frequencies (the highest peak in the left panel exceeds the scale) and the almost complete absence of spindles in other frequency ranges. It is a methodological artifact, reflecting properties of the applied MP algorithm [4], not the properties of the analyzed data. The right panel presents a histogram obtained from the same dataset using a bias-free implementation of MP in stochastic dictionaries [5].

If we are not sure whether the software we use for MP decompositions provides bias-free results, we may simply verify this issue by means of decomposing a large number of realizations of signals of exactly known properties, like white noise, and verifying the properties of MP decompositions, as presented in Figure 7.3 or Figure 13.1. Bias-free implementations of MP can be downloaded from http://signalml.org or http://eeg.pl/mp.

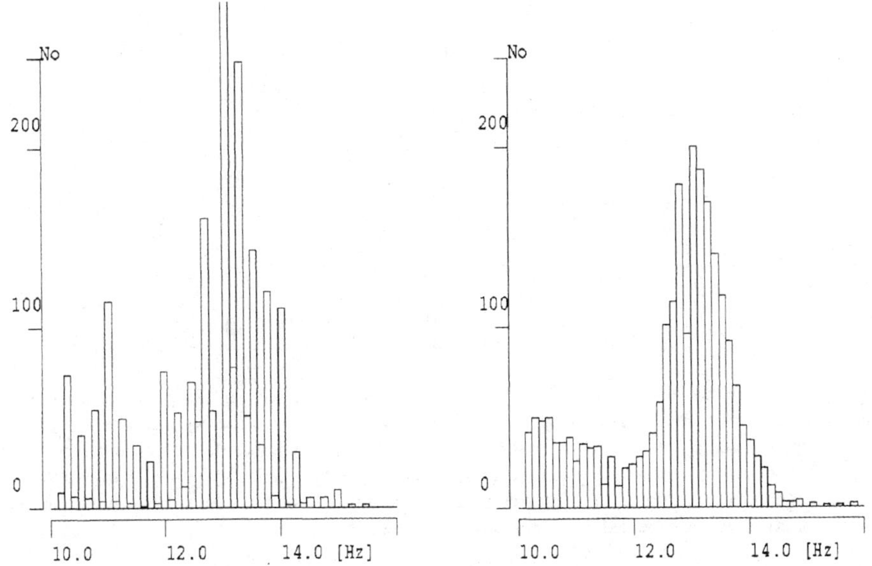

Figure 7.2 Frequency histograms of sleep spindles detected in derivation Pz of an overnight EEG recording (for details, see Section 8.2). The left panel presents results obtained from the mpp software package accompanying publication [4]. In the right panel—histogram obtained for the same EEG data from a bias-free implementation of MP in stochastic dictionaries [5].

7.4 LIMITATIONS OF GABOR DICTIONARIES

With properly chosen parameters, Gabor functions can match a wide variety of waveforms, as exemplified in Figure 5.2, but not all. For example, Plate 1 presents decomposition of a signal containing chirp (i.e., oscillation of linearly increasing frequency). Since Gabor dictionaries contain only waveforms of constant frequencies, a chirp cannot be concisely expressed by a single dictionary function. A partial workaround for representing time-frequency energy density of changing frequencies with a Gabor dictionary is presented in Figure 13.2. For special purposes it is possible to implement MP with dictionaries containing any other functions. But if we take these limitations into account when interpreting the results, in most cases Gabor dictionaries are enough.

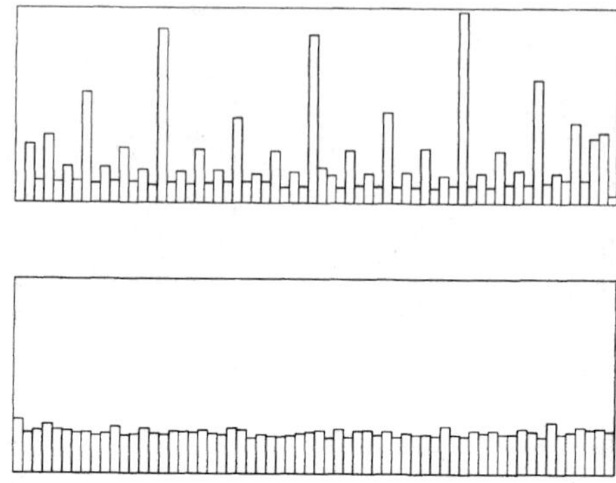

Figure 7.3 Frequency histograms of MP decompositions of 200 epochs of 128-point realizations of white noise. The horizontal axis corresponds to frequency (from zero to the Nyquist frequency), the vertical axis represents the number of cases. The histogram in the upper panel was obtained from implementation accompanying [4] and reflects the structure of the dictionary rather than that of the decomposed data. The histogram in the lower panel was obtained from MP with stochastic dictionaries [5] and approximates the expected flat distribution in frequencies.

References

[1] C. de Vleeschouwer and A. Zakhor, "In-Loop Atom Modulus Quantization for Matching Pursuit and Its Application to Video Coding," *IEEE Transactions on Image Processing*, vol. 12, no. 10, October 2003, pp. 1226–1242.

[2] R. Neff and A. Zakhor, "Modulus Quantization for Matching Pursuit Video Coding," *IEEE Transactions on Circuits and Systems for Video Technology*, vol. 10, no. 6, January 2000, pp. 13–26.

[3] R. Norcen, P. Schneider, and A. Uhl, "Approaching Real-Time Processing for Matching Pursuit Image Coding," *Media Processors 2002*, S. Panchanathan, V. Bove, and S. I. Sudharsanan, (eds.), vol. 4674 of *SPIE Proceedings*, 2002, pp. 84–90.

[4] S. Mallat and Z. Zhang, "Matching Pursuit with Time-Frequency Dictionaries," *IEEE Transactions on Signal Processing*, vol. 41, December 1993, pp. 3397–3415.

[5] P. J. Durka, D. Ircha, and K. J. Blinowska, "Stochastic Time-Frequency Dictionaries for Matching Pursuit," *IEEE Transactions on Signal Processing*, vol. 49, no. 3, March 2001, pp. 507–510.

Part II

EEG Analysis

Chapter 8

Parameterization of EEG Transients

After a brief introduction of electroencephalography, this chapter gathers results related to the parametric description of structures, known from visual EEG analysis, in terms of waveforms fitted to the signal by the MP algorithm. A universal framework is developed and then applied to sleep EEG structures and epileptic events. This framework can be easily adopted to any transients, definable in terms of time-frequency parameters.

"Animal electricity" has been subject to scientific research since the end of the eighteenth century, when Galvani and Volta performed their famous experiments [1]. Electrical activity of the brain was first mentioned in 1875, in a grant report by Caton [2]. The first electroencephalogram (EEG) was recorded from the surface of a human skull by Berger in 1929 [3].

The year 1935 witnessed the birth of the major fields of today's clinical electroencephalography. Gibbs and Davis [4] showed association of 3/second spike-wave complexes in EEG with epileptic petit mal absences, and Loomis et al. [5] methodically studied human sleep EEG patterns and the stages of sleep. Also in 1935, the first electroencephalograph (Grass Model I) started the era of contemporary EEG recording: galvanometers, used in earlier decades to record EEG traces on photographic paper, were replaced by three-channel preamplifiers, and the recordings were drawn by ink writers on rolls of paper. These rolls were later replaced by folded paper, and, currently, by digital storage and display of EEG traces. Also, contemporary amplifiers provide higher sensitivity and number of channels, but all these changes are quantitative rather than qualitative.

Finally, by the end of 1940s, Dawson [6] recorded the first evoked potentials. Later he constructed an advanced mechano-electrical (analog) device for averaging brains potentials triggered by a stimulus [7]. Averaging was indispensable to show the event-related activity, which is normally invisible in the ongoing EEG background (Figure 8.1).

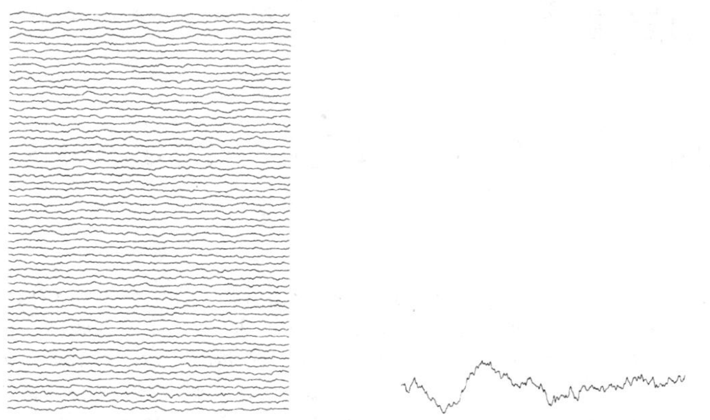

Figure 8.1 Left: fifty-five 1-second EEG traces. These epochs were selected from a continuous recording of wake EEG in a way that the beginning of each 1-second epoch is aligned in time with an occurrence of a randomly repeated audio stimulus. Right: their plain average. The vertical scale is enhanced to present the components of an auditory evoked potential. For example, the largest positive hump is known as P300. This is a positive deflection of the voltage occurring approximately 300 ms from the onset of an unexpected stimulus (the whole epoch lasts 1 second).

To the present day, EEG is being used continuously in clinical practice. On the technological side, there was an obvious improvement in recording and storage of the signal. This progress has reached certain saturation in terms of satisfying accuracy and number of derivations recorded simultaneously. Unfortunately, the progress in the methodology of analysis of these huge amounts of valuable data, especially in clinical applications, seems to be incomparably slower.

First applications of signal processing methods to EEG can be traced back to 1932, when Berger and Dietsch applied Fourier analysis to short EEG sections [8]. Then, quoting [9]:

> The 1950s saw the early generation of automatic frequency analyzers approaching and eventually saw the end of these magnificent but mostly unused machines.

Digital storage of EEG time series greatly facilitated the application of signal processing methods, as well as any other mathematical analysis. In spite of this, after 75 years, clinical EEG analysis still relies almost exclusively on visual inspection of raw EEG traces. Advanced mathematical methods are being widely applied in basic neurophysiological research, but not in clinical practice. This situation is reflected in the report of the American Academy of Neurology and the American Clinical Neurophysiology Society [10], which explicitly discourages application of signal processing methods in clinical practice (except as auxiliary tools). Therefore, the only significant change in the clinical EEG analysis is summarized in Figure 8.2: visual analysis of paper recordings was replaced by visual analysis of digital recordings displayed on computer screen.

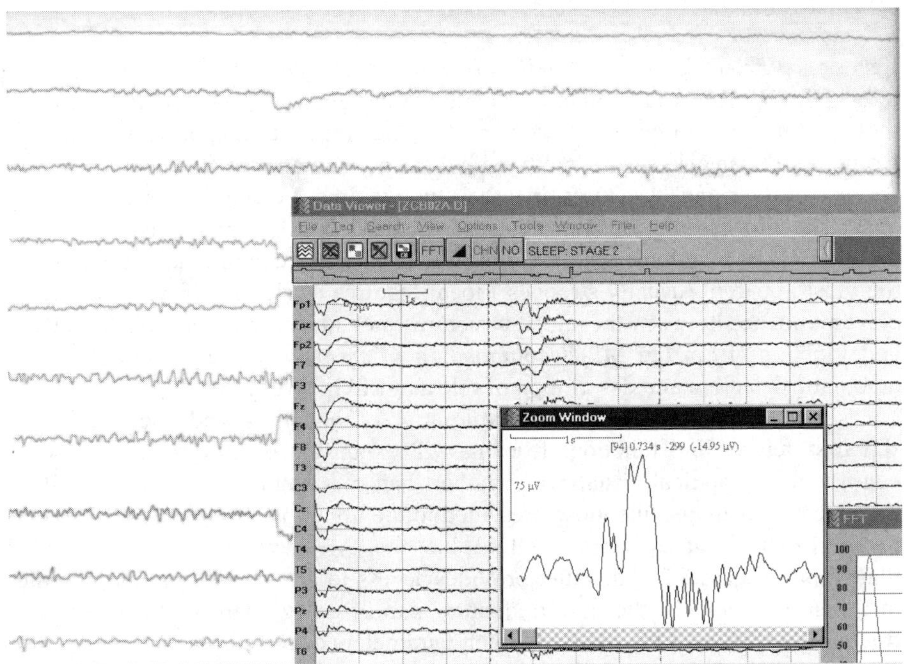

Figure 8.2 Seventy years of progress in clinical electroencephalography: from visual analysis of EEG traces on paper (background picture) to visual analysis of EEG traces displayed on CRT (front). (*From:* [11]. © 2001 IEEE. Reprinted with permission.)

In the following sections we will explore the possibilities of establishing a direct correspondence between advanced signal processing and visual EEG analysis. Such a link would be extremely beneficial for both clinical and research applications of EEG. Reliable automatization of certain tedious tasks performed by skilled electroencephalographers would decrease the costs and increase the repeatability (and hence also reliability) of clinical EEG analysis. This correspondence may provide a direct access to the knowledge base of clinical and behavioral correlates, gathered over decades of visual EEG analysis. Such a link is essential for coherent progress in basic neuroscience research. If new hypotheses are formulated using incompatible terms, the huge intersubject variability usually calls for their verification on impractically large groups of subjects.

8.1 SELECTING RELEVANT STRUCTURES

Let us recall from Section 6.1 that the primary output of the MP algorithm is given in terms of parameters of the functions, fitted to the signal. As presented in Figure 6.1, these parameters can be used to construct a time-frequency map of energy density. However, we can also work directly with these parameters, which describe physical features of the signal structures, like their time widths and amplitudes.

The process of visual analysis of an EEG epoch is partly similar to the function of the matching pursuit algorithm. The human eye first naturally fixes on the most apparent (usually strongest) local features of signals. If we could find a correspondence between the signal structures picked by electroencephalographers and functions from the MP decomposition of the signal, we could achieve an automatic detection and description of relevant EEG waveforms.

For the first experiences with exploration of the correspondence between the signal structures and functions from its MP expansion, it may be convenient to begin with a graphical visualization rather than raw numbers. We may use static time-frequency maps, like those presented in the upper panel of Figure 6.1, Figure 8.4, and Plate 3, or an interactive tool, like the "MPview" program presented in Plate 2 and Figure 8.3. The latter provides access to all the information presented in Figure 6.1, not just the time-frequency map of energy density. For each time-frequency blob under the mouse pointer, parameters of the corresponding function are displayed in the lower right corner. For a blob selected by clicking the mouse on its center, the time course of the corresponding function (such as those presented in the middle panels of Figure 6.1) is added to the reconstruction signal, plotted under the time-frequency map.

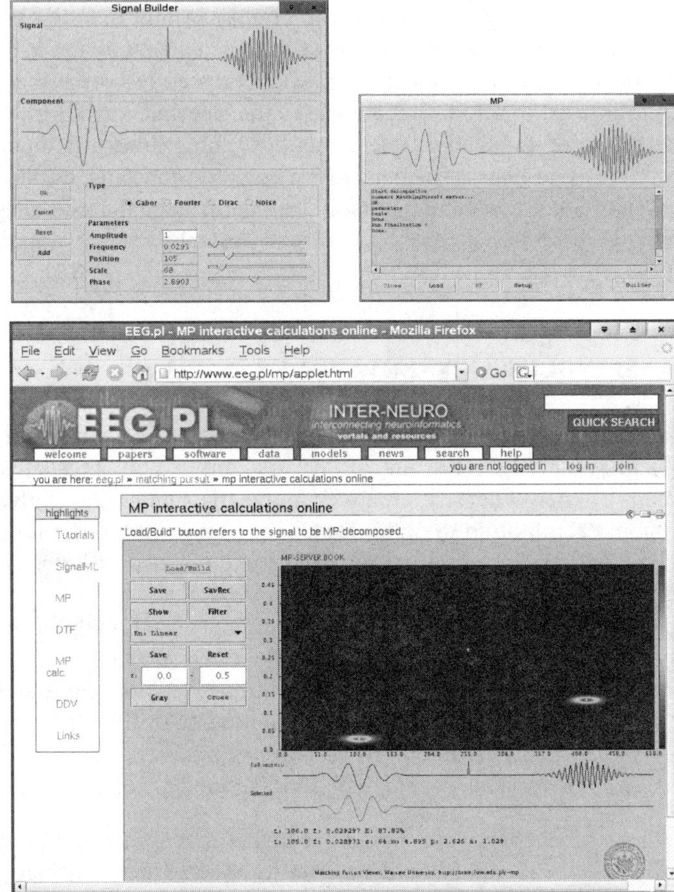

Figure 8.3 Online version of the MPview program from Plate 2, with an option to run MP decompositions. Web interface is accessible via the "MP calc." option from the left tab in the eeg.pl portal. Clicking the "Load/Build" button opens the window presented in the upper-right panel, which allows us to read an ASCII signal from local disk or to build a simulated signal (the "Builder" window shown in the upper-left panel). Parameters of the decomposition can be adjusted after clicking the "Setup" button. After completing the decomposition, we are returned to the main window with the time-frequency map, calculated from this decomposition, which can be explored interactively just like the program from Plate 2. Written by D. Ircha (dobi@message.pl).

In such a way we may gain a first exploratory insight into a possible correspondence between the functions fitted to the analyzed signal by the MP procedure and the structures of interest, visible in the raw EEG traces. However, there is also an a priori path to this exploration: in many cases the relevant waveforms are at least approximately defined in standardized terms describing their prominent features, like amplitude (peak to peak), frequency (cycles per second), or duration in time. As a unique feature of the matching pursuit[1] among the signal processing methods, these features can be simultaneously and directly matched to the language of MP decomposition.

8.2 SLEEP SPINDLES AND SLOW WAVES

Figure 8.4 and Plate 3 exemplify MP parameterization of some typical transients from sleep and wake EEG. Results of MP decomposition, presented as time-frequency maps of energy density, are given above the signals. As explained in the previous section, each blob in the time-frequency plane relates to a function from the MP decomposition. Each of these functions is described in terms of time and frequency positions, time width, amplitude, and phase.

The paradigm, which gives a hope of bridging visual analysis of EEG and advanced signal processing, is surprisingly simple. It was first applied in mid-1990s for detection of sleep spindles, since these structures reveal the shape closest to the Gabor functions (i.e., waxing and waning oscillations). In the classical reference *A manual of standardized terminology, techniques and scoring system for sleep stages in human subjects* [12], sleep spindles are defined as follows:

> The presence of sleep spindle should not be defined unless it is of at least 0.5 sec duration, i.e., one should be able to count 6 or 7 distinct waves within the half-second period. [...] The term should be used only to describe activity between 12 and 14 cps.

Such a definition can be directly translated into the language of the parameters of the waveforms fitted to the signal by the matching pursuit algorithm, to obtain a possible one-to-one correspondence between the sleep spindles seen by the electroencephalographers and Gabor functions selected from the MP decomposition of corresponding EEG traces. To explore this correspondence, a filter was constructed to select from the MP decompositions of sleep EEG those structures

1 Strictly speaking, it is a feature of the adaptive time-frequency approximations, and matching pursuit is currently the only implementation available for practical applications.

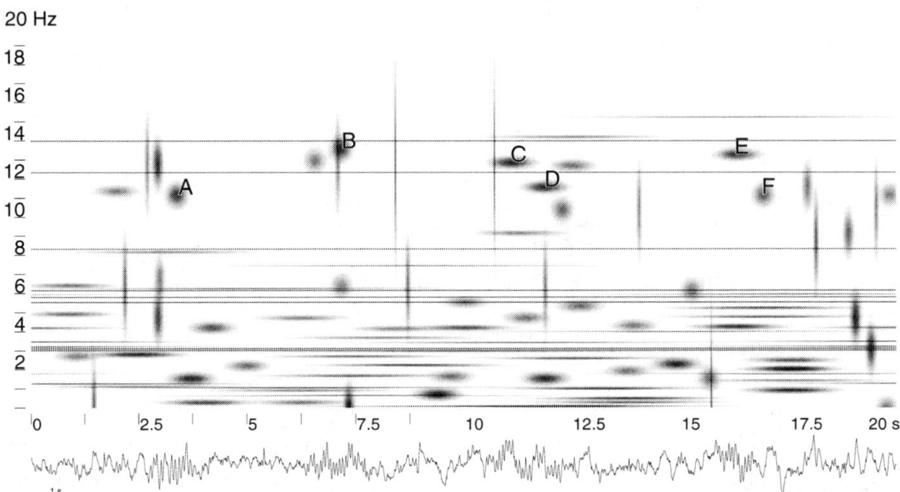

Figure 8.4 Time-frequency distribution of energy density of 20 seconds of sleep EEG; structures corresponding to sleep spindles are marked by letters A–F. Structures C and D, as well as E and F, were classified as one spindle (i.e., their centers fell within a time section marked by an expert as one spindle) [13].

that correspond to sleep spindles, based upon the following criteria: frequency from 11 to 15 Hz,[2] time duration from 0.5 to 2.5 seconds, and amplitude above 25 μV. Direct application of this filter gives an automatic detection and parameterization of all the structures—conforming to these criteria—that are present in the analyzed recordings. We may expect that these structures correspond to the sleep spindles as perceived by electroencephalographers.

Confirmation of such expectations and necessary adjustments is a tedious and complicated task, partly addressed in the next section. Among many practical problems, some discrepancies were also caused by superimposed spindles, like the cases marked C/D and E/F in Figure 8.4. Nevertheless, the expected correspondence was achieved and confirmed [13, 14]. Similarly, criteria for detecting slow waves were formulated based upon [12]; agreement of the automatic parameterization of slow waves with visual detection was confirmed a posteriori a few years later in [15].

2 The classical 12–14-Hz frequency range of sleep spindles, defined originally in [12], was later considered too narrow.

Ranges of parameters, used for the automatic selection of delta waves and sleep spindles from the MP decompositions of sleep EEG, are given in Table 8.1.

Table 8.1

Criteria Defining Sleep Spindles and Slow Waves, Used in Figures 8.5 and 8.6.

	Frequency	*Time Duration*	*Min. Amplitude*
Delta waves	0.5–4 Hz	0.5–∞ s.	75 μV
Sleep spindles	11–15 Hz	0.5–2.5 s.	15 μV

Source: [13].

Let us forget for a moment about the majority of problems inherent to the biomedical sciences. Suppose that definitions from Table 8.1 reflect perfectly some objective and consistent reality. In such a case we would achieve—by means of a simple and fully controllable algorithm—even more than a fully automatic detection of all the relevant structures in arbitrarily long recordings. Apart from the very detection, each of these structures is described in terms of its amplitude, frequency and time positions, duration, and phase. We can view this information as a database of relevant structures; from this database we can create reports, fitted to answer any well-posed question—that is, any question addressing the actual information content of the signal, related to these structures.

As an example, Figure 8.5 presents time courses of frequencies, amplitudes, and numbers of occurrences per minute, of all sleep spindles detected in 7 hours of sleep EEG. Similarly, amplitudes, frequencies, and average powers are plotted for delta waves. We appreciate the consistency of these reports with the classical description of the sleep process, represented by the manually constructed hypnogram, plotted in the same time scale in the upper panel. In agreement with the experience gained in decades of visual analysis (and with the definitions of sleep stages [12]), we observe the absence of sleep spindles in REM periods, increased slow wave activity in the deep sleep stages (3 and 4), and the reciprocal relation between the appearance of sleep spindles and slow waves. All these conclusions are clearly summarized in a single picture, constructed from a precise and automatic parameterization of all the relevant structures, which can be used directly for statistical evaluation of hypotheses.

Reports from the databases describing relevant structures, selected from the MP decomposition, are by no means limited to a single channel of EEG. Available recordings often contain several channels—for example, the 10–20 international

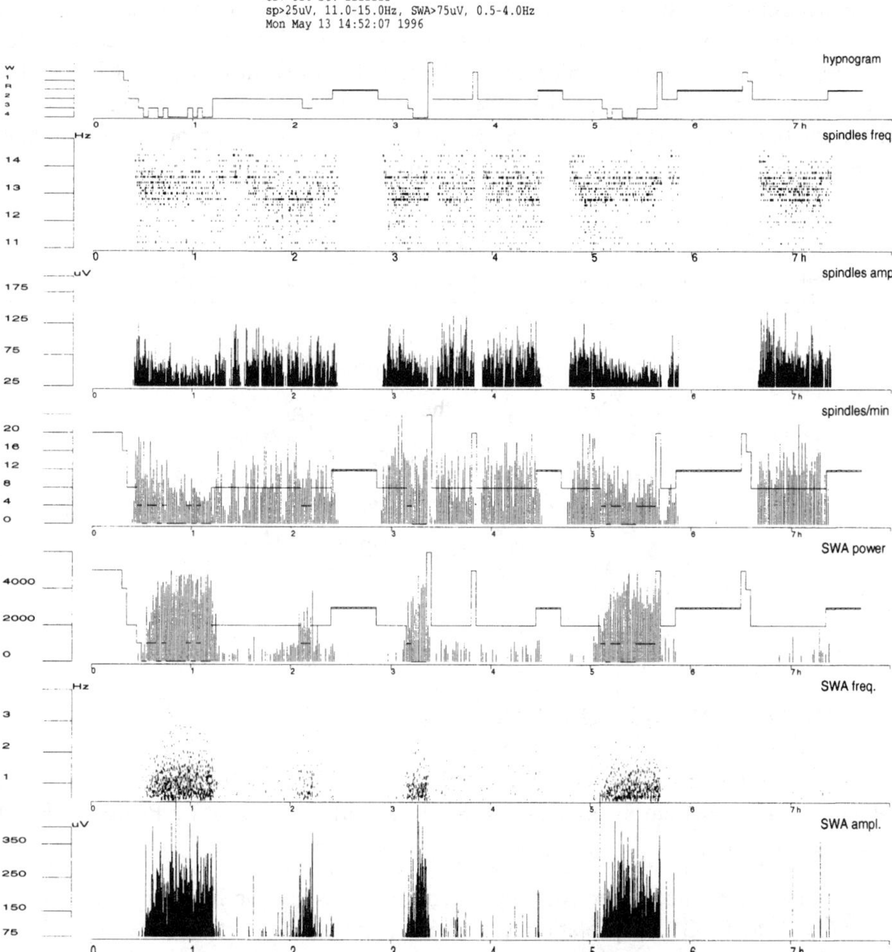

Figure 8.5 Upper plot: hypnogram constructed by an experienced electroencephalographer. Following, in the same time scale, the results of automatic detection of sleep spindles and slow waves, using MP decomposition of EEG from electrode Pz and filters from Table 8.1. From the top: frequencies, amplitudes, and number of occurrences per minute of sleep spindles. Lower three plots: average power per minute, frequencies, and amplitudes of slow waves. We can observe absence of sleep spindles in the REM periods and the reciprocal relations between spindling activity and SWA [13].

standard defines positions of 21 electrodes (Table 8.2). A complete evaluation of the relations between signal structures recorded in different electrodes requires solving so-called inverse problem for EEG, which will be discussed in Chapter 12. Nevertheless, for now we can visualize the results of separate decompositions of all the available signals as in Figure 8.6. But before we continue exploration of the new possibilities opened by this approach, we must first consider some caveats.

Table 8.2

Relative Positions of Electrodes in 10–20 System, Front of Head Toward the Top of Page

	Fp1	Fpz	Fp2	
F7	F3	Fz	F4	F8
T3	C3	Cz	C4	T4
T5	P3	Pz	P4	T6
	O1	Oz	O2	

8.3 REAL-WORLD PROBLEMS

These problems are the reason this book was written in 2006 rather than 1996, when results presented in Figures 8.4–8.6 were obtained. Quoting Professor Ernst Niedermayer [16]:

> Every experienced electroencephalographer has his or her personal approach to EEG interpretation. [...] there is an element of science and element of art in a good EEG interpretation; it is the latter that defies standardization.

It is a very elegant way of introducing the inherent limitations of visual analysis, but no matter how we say it, the fact remains the same: given low repeatability of the visual analysis, reflected in the limited interexpert agreement,[3] it is not easy to turn this art into a science, which by definition relies on reproducible experiments.

3 Lack of a strict repeatability is not only reflected in limited accordance between experts. Limited repeatability of the same experts' decisions in a double-blind test was reported, for example, in [18].

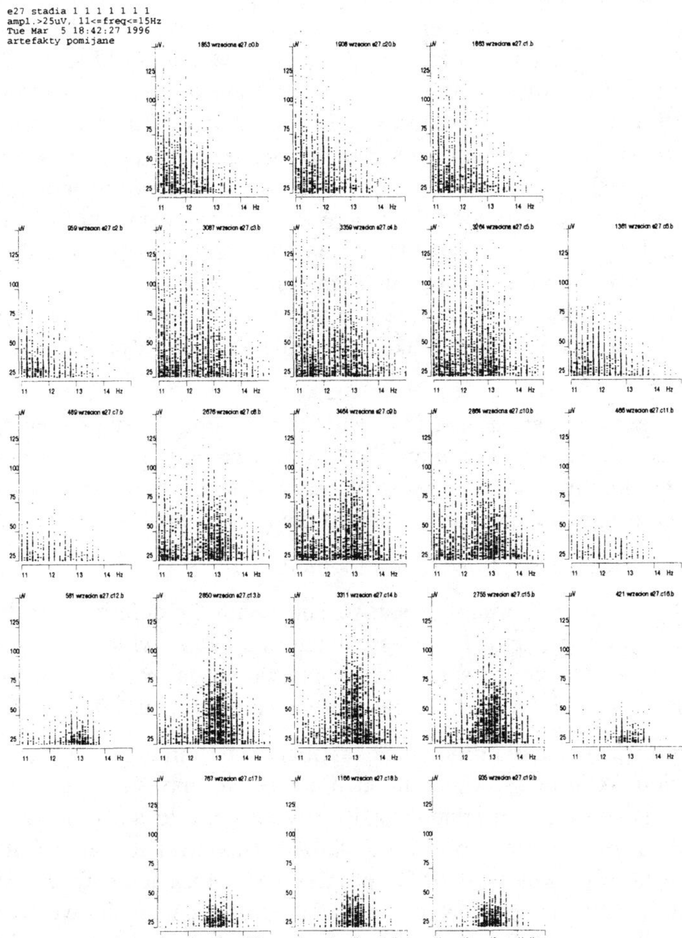

Figure 8.6 Sleep spindles detected in 21 derivations of overnight sleep, decomposed separately. Each spindle is marked as a small cross in frequency (horizontal, Hz) versus amplitude (vertical, μV) coordinates. Plots are organized topographically according to the relative positions of electrodes (Table 8.2), top of the head upwards. We observe prevalence of lower frequencies in frontal, and higher frequencies in parietal derivations [13]. Also, some frequencies appear more often—this statistical bias, present in a fast implementation of MP [17], will be discussed in Section 13.8.

For example, the main reference [12] defines slow waves as structures of amplitude above 75 μV. However, it is generally acknowledged that variable skull thickness [19], age and sex differences [20, 21], and quality of sleep [22] can influence the overall amplitude of EEG. Therefore, an experienced electroencephalographer instinctively lowers the threshold of slow waves' amplitude in case of a generally lower EEG amplitude observed in the whole recording. A nearly linear relation between the mean amplitude of the whole EEG recording and the minimum slow wave amplitude assumed by electroencephalographers marking sleep stages according to [12] was suggested in [15]. The same problem relates to the minimum amplitude of sleep spindles or any other structures.

But the situation is even more difficult for structures lacking a priori definitions in time-frequency terms, like K-complexes. Let us quote again the basic reference [12]:

> K complexes are defined as EEG wave forms having a well delineated negative sharp wave which is immediately followed by a positive component. The total duration of the complex should exceed 0.5 sec. Waves of 12–14 cps may or may not constitute a part of the K complex.

This text is immediately followed by a footnote:

> This definition of K complex is at variance with the definition of the Terminology Committee of the International Federation which is as follows: "Combination of vertex sharp waves and sigma paroxysm, occurring simultaneously and especially in response to sudden stimuli during sleep."

Obviously, such a definition is not applicable within the framework presented in the previous section. However, in such a case we may still use an a posteriori setting. It consists of determining the MP correlates of relevant structures by means of comparison of the decompositions of the signal with the visual markings of human experts. But in the case of K-complexes, even the interexpert agreement in their visual detection is very low (e.g., in [23], 50% agreement between two experts is reported). We will briefly recall the issue of K-complexes in Section 8.5.

These examples provide only a small sample of the problems related to the limited repeatability of visual EEG analysis and the lack of strict definitions of relevant structures, waveforms, and rhythms. In the last decade, several studies (e.g., [11, 14, 15, 24–26]) were dedicated to finding partial solutions within the framework discussed in this book. Their results indicate that in most cases we should be able to achieve agreement of the MP-based detection with the visual analysis on the level, similar to the interexpert accordance in detection of given structures.

8.4 HYPNOGRAM AND CONTINUOUS DESCRIPTION OF SLEEP

Let us recall the hypnogram, which we encountered in the upper panel of Figure 8.5 (another example is presented in the upper panel of Figure 8.7). It represents the standard interpretation of polysomnographic recordings,[4] which relies on a division into sleep stages, assigned to 20- or 30-second long epochs. Criteria defining sleep stages were summarized by Rechtschaffen and Kales in 1968 [12]. In particular, definitions of sleep stages 3 and 4 rely mainly on the content of slow waves:

> Stage 3 is defined by an EEG record in which at least 20% but not more than 50% of the epoch consists of waves of 2 cps or slower which have amplitudes greater than 75 μV peak to peak [...]
>
> Stage 4 is defined by an EEG record in which more than 50% of the epoch consists of waves of 2 cps or slower [...]

These definitions relate to the visual analysis of EEG. Can we apply them directly in the framework of contemporary signal processing?

As presented in Figure 3.12, spectral methods of signal analysis do not provide information on the time extent of the frequencies appearing in the spectrum. Likewise, time-frequency methods like spectrogram, wavelets, or Wigner-like transforms, mentioned in Chapter 4, do not return explicitly time durations of the oscillations appearing in the signal. This magnitude might be estimated from some postprocessing of time-frequency transforms, but given the dependence of their resolutions on particular arbitrary settings—like the width of the analysis window in spectrogram, the smoothing kernel for Wigner transform, or different choices of wavelets—these estimates would be neither reliable nor high resolution.

Matching pursuit is the first general method that explicitly approximates the time span of each oscillation detected in a signal.[5] Once we set the criteria for waveforms considered slow waves, in each subsequent 20-second epoch we can easily compute the percentage of the interval they occupy. Time course of this percentage is presented in the middle panel of Figure 8.7. The upper panel presents a

4 Polysomnogram is a recording of EEG and other signals—like muscle activity (electromyogram, EMG), eye movement (electrooculogram, ECoG), heart electric activity (electrocardiogram, ECG), and breathing rate—during sleep.

5 Strictly speaking, it is the time span of the dictionary's function, chosen to represent a given waveform—actually the half-width of the Gaussian envelope—so the estimate is most accurate when the amplitude of the oscillation is modulated by Gaussian. In the standard time-frequency dictionaries, we have only constant frequencies, so this remark does not relate to structures of varying frequency.

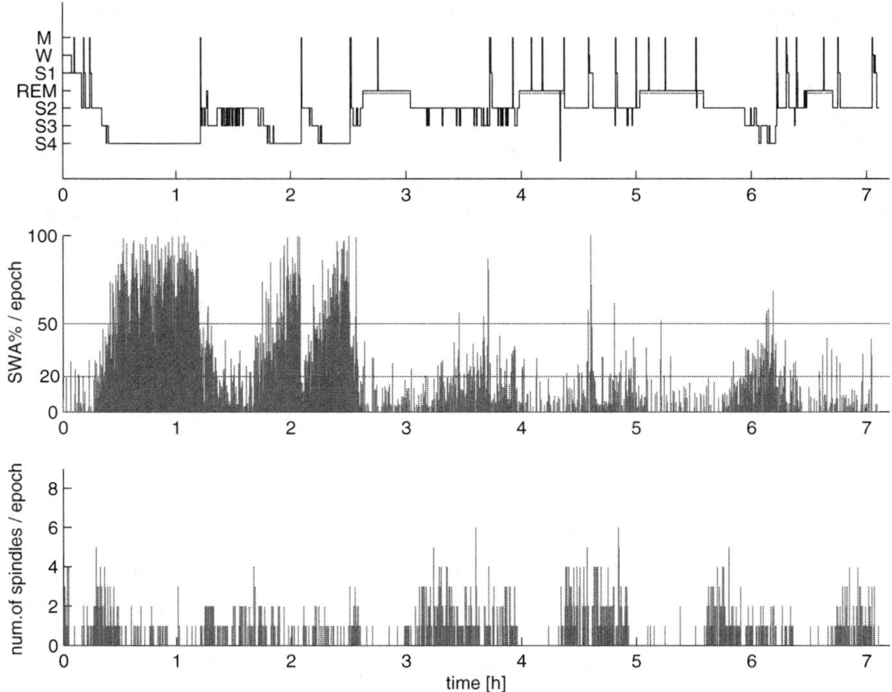

Figure 8.7 Top: hypnogram (by human expert); bottom: SWA and sleep spindles detected automatically; % SWA denotes the percentage of the epoch's time occupied by waveforms classified as SWA. This continuous description of the slow wave sleep is fully compatible with the classification of stages 3/4 by Rechtschaffen and Kales [12], as indicated by the 20% and 50% lines. Artifacts not removed from analysis. (Reprinted from [15]. © 2005, with permission from Elsevier.)

hypnogram, scored for the same EEG record by an experienced electroencephalographer. We observe a very good agreement of the ratio of time occupied by slow waves in each epoch with the 20% and 50% limits, related to the previously quoted definitions of stages 3 and 4, and visually scored hypnogram.

Let us contemplate Figure 8.7 in a wider context. Description of sleep in terms of stages assigned to epochs of fixed width, defined by Rechtschaffen and Kales in [12], is being continuously criticized. New descriptors, often difficult to reproduce, are being proposed in contradiction with the parsimony principle. Nevertheless, classical staging to the present day remains the only common description used in both clinical and research applications of polysomnograms. Among constructive critics, the need for a finer time scale and a measure of spindle intensity was suggested in [27]. Both these needs are easily satisfied in a simple report from the database of sleep spindles and slow waves, presented in Figure 8.7.

A continuous description of the slow wave sleep was already presented in the lower panels of Figure 8.5; another continuous estimator can be computed in terms of spectral integrals, as presented in Figure 8.8. But Figure 8.7 shows unambiguously that the description of slow wave sleep based upon the MP parameterization of relevant structures is also fully compatible with the previous approach (i.e., staging) established in almost four decades of worldwide applications. The classical deep sleep stages 3 and 4 appear as a direct simplification of this approach; it can be viewed as application of fixed 20% and 50% thresholds to the plot from the middle panel of Figure 8.7, which reflects the continuous nature of sleep. Detailed comparison of this approach with visual staging is discussed in [15].

As presented in Figure 8.8, estimators of spindling and slow wave activities can be computed simply as spectral integrals in sigma and delta bands. However, as discussed previously, such estimators do not provide direct information on the time occupied by the relevant structures. Also, as clearly visible in the head-to-head comparison in Figure 8.8, spectral estimates incorporate a significant amount of noise. Adaptive parameterization of relevant structures allows for construction of much more sensitive estimators than the spectral integrals. When computing the spectral integrals, from all the information contained in Table 8.1 we can use only the frequency limits of the corresponding bands, while MP-based estimates also employ thresholds on time widths and amplitudes of relevant structures. Selectivity of MP-based estimates of energy is discussed further in Chapter 11.

8.5 SENSITIVITY TO PHASE AND FREQUENCY

In Section 8.3 we mentioned problems related to the ambiguous definition of K-complexes and limited repeatability of their visual detection. These issues cannot be solved by a purely mathematical approach. However, sensitivity of the matching pursuit algorithm to phase and frequency of the oscillations present in the signal can facilitate differentiation of K-complexes from a background containing slow activity.

Waveforms of similar time-frequency signatures are very difficult to distinguish using the classical time-frequnecy methods. On the contrary, matching pursuit algorithm is very sensitive to small differences in either frequency or phase: continuous oscillations will be broken down into a series of separate structures in the

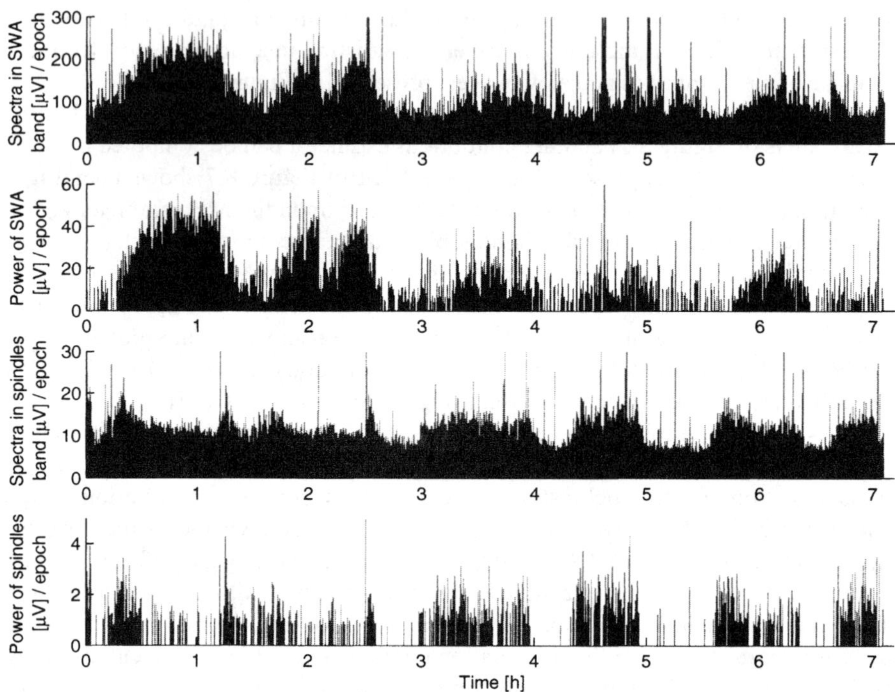

Figure 8.8 Top: square root of the power of SWA, calculated from spectral integrals in ranges corresponding to Table 8.1 and power of SWA estimated for structures detected in the MP decomposition. Bottom: the same for sleep spindles. Power is in sqrt scale, time of the sleep is in hours. As in Figure 8.7, artifact-contaminated epochs are not removed to preserve the continuity of time. (Reprinted from [15]. © 2005, with permission from Elsevier.)

presence of subtle changes in frequency or phase. If we assume that the activity of a single structure generates activity of constant phase, this effect may be helpful in distinguishing signal structures related to the activities of different generators, and hence also to different physiological phenomena.

Figure 8.9 gives an example of a K-complex, which is hard to distinguish by eye from the ongoing slow wave activity. However, due to subtle differences in phase and frequency, it is parameterized by the MP algorithm as a separate structure. Unfortunately, because of difficulties related to the low interexpert concordance in detection of K-complexes, discussed in Section 8.3, an efficient detection and parameterization of K-complexes is still one of the open issues.

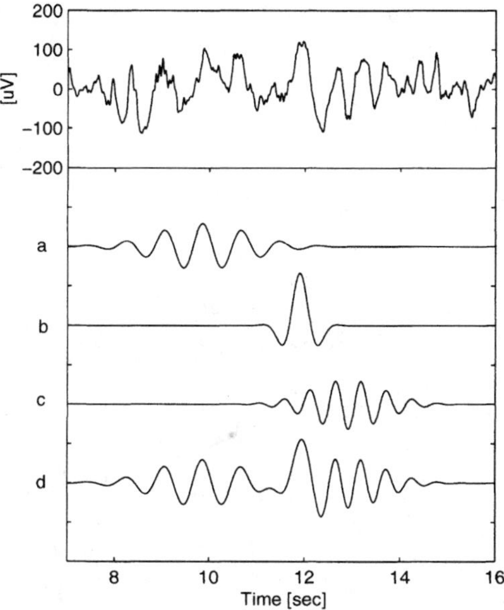

Figure 8.9 Example of a slow wave activity, containing a single K-complex that is not phase-locked to the SWA. Therefore, in the MP parameterization it appears as a separate structure, giving a reliable distinction between the synchronized slow waves and a separate, nonsynchronized structure. At the top is the original signal, the middle shows the waveforms from the Gabor dictionary that represent some components of decreasing energy: (a) and (c) correspond to slow wave activity, while (b) corresponds to a structure marked by a clinician as K-complex. Bottom trace (d) presents superposition of waveforms (a) to (c). (*From:* [28]. © 2006 IEEE. Reprinted with permission.)

8.6 NONOSCILLATING STRUCTURES

Let us recall that dictionaries used for matching pursuit decomposition of signals are usually constructed from Gabor functions (i.e., sinusoidal oscillations modulated by Gaussian envelope). K-complex from Figure 8.9 at a first glance can be hardly classified as a Gabor function. However, already in Figure 5.2 we may have noticed that the variety of possible shapes of the Gabor functions also includes significant variations from the purity of waxing and waning oscillations, confined to a clearly distinguishable Gaussian envelope. These variations occur in cases when the period of the oscillation is similar to the width of the envelope. Denoting the period of the oscillation as $T = \frac{2\pi}{\omega}$, and the width of the envelope as s, this is equivalent to $T \approx s$ or $\omega s \approx 2\pi$.

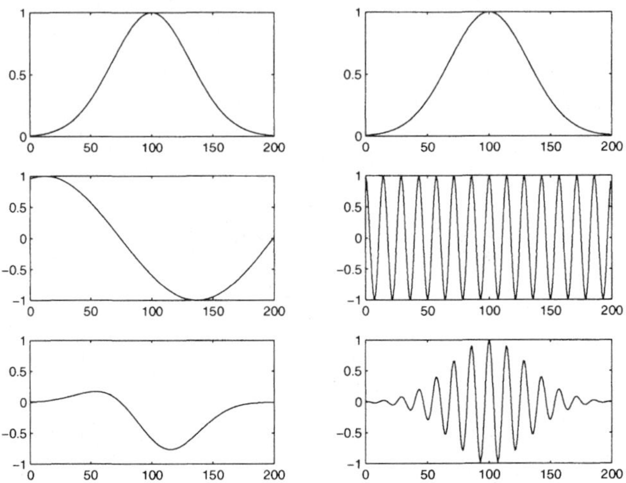

Figure 8.10 Two Gabor functions created from the same Gaussian envelope (upper row) and different frequencies of modulating sines (middle row). The bottom row shows Gabor functions as a product of the above. In the left column the width of the Gaussian is similar to the period of the sine.

Figure 8.10 explains the genesis of such cases by presenting separately the Gaussian envelope (upper row, the same for both cases) and the sinusoidal oscillations (middle row). Their products constitute Gabor functions, presented in the lower row. The right column presents a "classical" case, where the sinusoidal oscillation is clearly distinguishable from the Gaussian envelope. In such a case, we may easily outline the time course of the Gaussian envelope and measure the period[6] of oscillations, also in the lower plot presenting their product.

On the contrary, for the case presented in the left column, the shapes of both these components are similar; therefore, it is difficult to distinguish in their product (lower plot) which feature (hump) of the resulting Gabor function is due to the oscillation and which to the envelope. Also, for the low-frequency modulation, presented in the left column, both the effective peak-to-peak amplitude and the visually perceived width of the structure are smaller. Figure 8.11 presents time-frequency density of energy of the two structures composed in Figure 8.10.

6 Or, equivalently, the frequency, since $f = \frac{1}{T}$.

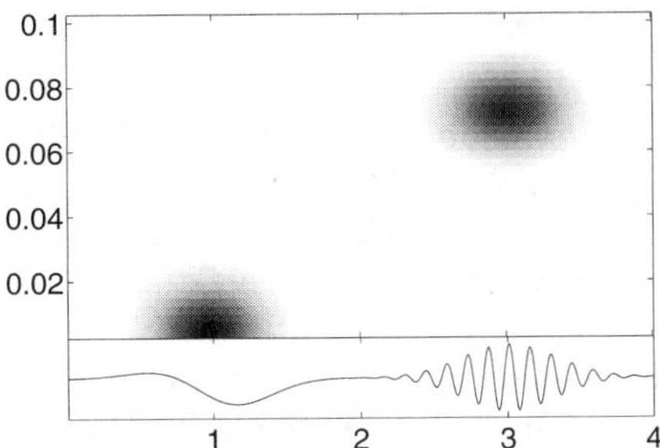

Figure 8.11 Time-frequency energy density of a simulated signal, composed from the two Gabor functions constructed in Figure 8.10.

For such nonoscillating or weakly oscillating structures, present in the electroencephalographic time series, the traditional description involved different terms than those used for clear oscillations. These differences can be observed, for example, by comparing the definitions of a sleep spindle (quoted on page 68) and K-complex (page 74). Nevertheless, all these waveforms can be efficiently described within the framework of adaptive time-frequency approximations in Gabor dictionaries. Such a universal and unifying approach is especially valuable in cases that are hard to classify a priori as oscillating or nonoscillating.

The differences between these two types of structures must be taken into account when investigating relations between the parameters of Gabor functions and the properties of waveforms perceived visually. In particular, for the standard, clearly oscillating waveforms—like the one in the left column of Figure 8.10—the doubled[7] amplitude of the Gabor envelope is equivalent to the peak-to-peak amplitude (that is, the difference between the highest and the lowest point of the function) of the resulting Gabor function. But comparison of the two lower panels of Figure 8.10 reveals that for nonoscillating structures, the peak-to-peak amplitude may be significantly less than double the amplitude of the Gabor envelope. Also, the effective width of such a function may be lower than the width of the envelope. The following chapter presents ways we can correct for these factors in practice.

7 The Gaussian envelope modulates sine, ranging from -1 to 1. Therefore, if the Gaussian has a unit amplitude, then the minimum value of the Gabor function will be -1, the maximum will be 1, and peak-to-peak amplitude will be 2.

8.7 EPILEPTIC EEG SPIKES

Since the discovery made by Gibbs and Davis in 1935 [4], epilepsy is one of the major fields of application of EEG. The next chapter is devoted entirely to the analysis of epileptic seizures. In this section we address the detection of epileptic spikes (see Figure 8.12), present in interictal EEG, that is, occurring in between the seizures.

The traditional definition of a spike is based on terms like amplitude, duration, sharpness, and emergence from the background. The first two terms, just like in the case of sleep EEG transients, are directly translatable into the parameters of the functions fitted by the MP algorithm. Therefore, the framework presented in the previous chapters can be applied for their parameterization and detection. However, in this case we must take into account the discrepancies between mathematical parameters of Gabor functions and physical features of waveforms, discussed in the previous section. For waveforms that have widths similar to the period of the modulation ($\omega s \approx 2\pi$), parameters of the Gabor functions [g_γ from Equation (13.16)] may describe the physical features of given structure (amplitude, half-width) rather indirectly. Nevertheless, the function g_γ, fitted to the given structure by the algorithm, still has the time course (shape) representing well the structure (if the structure is coherent with the applied dictionary). In such case we can retrieve the actual (effective) half-width and amplitude of the corresponding structure as the half-width of the extremum of g_γ and $\max(g_\gamma) - \min(g_\gamma)$, respectively.

In a pilot study [26], functions for which less than 1.5 periods of the sine modulation fits within the half-width of the Gabor envelope were treated as non-oscillating. For these structures, effective widths and amplitudes of Gabor functions fitted by the MP algorithm were calculated numerically to represent the physical widths and peak-to-peak amplitudes of the corresponding structures.

Once we are satisfied with the relevance of the parameters returned by the procedure, we can implement basically the same detection scheme, described in previous sections for sleep spindles and slow waves. Detection of spikes was performed by choosing from the structures fitted to the signal those conforming to a priori chosen parameters: half-width of the structure from 3 to 6 milliseconds and amplitude above 300 a.u.[8] These ranges of parameters were based upon the observed characteristics of structures designated as epileptic spikes in the visual analysis. Apart from this, a simple test was added to check whether the waveform

8 Amplitude was processed in arbitrary units, since the conversion ratio (points/μV) was not given in [29]. If this multiplicative constant is known, which is the case in clinical analyses, we are dealing with amplitude expressed in μV.

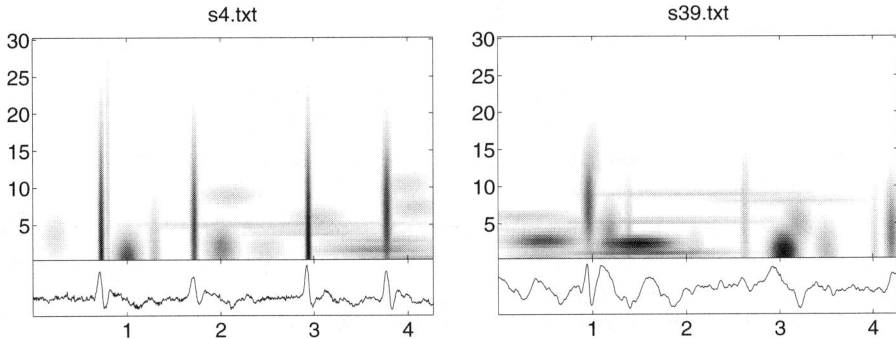

Figure 8.12 Time-frequency energy density of signals: the left panel contains four epileptic EEG spikes, the right panel contains a spike-wave complex occurring around the first second. The horizontal scale is in seconds, the vertical scale is in Hz. (Signals courtesy of authors of [29]. Reprinted figure with permission from [26]. © 2004 by the American Physical Society.)

was fitted to an edge of signal's step rather than a separate structure (i.e., local maximum), which was the case for some of the artifacts present in these data.

In such a way, we constructed a simple yet effective detector of epileptic spikes. It exhibited a very promising performance [26], which will have to be confirmed on larger datasets. For now let us stress two major advantages:

1. All parameters governing detection are expressed in terms directly related to the features perceived in visual analysis, which is the only reference for the automatic detectors. Therefore, the procedure can be fully understood, controlled, and tuned by those skilled in epileptology and the art of interpretation of EEG traces, and not necessarily in higher mathematics, required to understand the operation of a majority of other automatic detectors.

2. This approach relies on the same scheme and mathematical background as detection and description of other EEG waveforms presented in the previous sections. Such a unifying approach has obvious advantages in practical applications and conforms to the Occam's Razor, in terms of "not creating more descriptors than necessary."

Matlab scripts for performing the detection of spikes described in this section are available at http://eeg.pl. As a side effect of this study, another interesting feature of the matching pursuit decomposition was observed for series of spikes. It will be discussed in Section 9.1.

References

[1] A. N. Martonosi, "Animal Electricity, Ca^{2+} and Muscle Contraction. A Brief History of Muscle Research," *Acta Biochimica Polonica*, vol. 47, no. 3, 2000, pp. 493–516.

[2] M. A. B. Brazier, *A History of the Electrical Activity of the Brain: The First Half-Century*, London: Pitman Medical Publishing, 1961.

[3] H. Berger, "Über das Elektrenkephalogramm des Menschen," *Arch. f. Psychiat.*, vol. 87, 1929, pp. 527–570.

[4] F. A. Gibbs and H. Davis, "Changes in the Human Electroencephalogram Associated with Loss of Consciousness," *Am. J. Physiol.*, vol. 113, 1935, pp. 49–50.

[5] A. L. Loomis, E. N. Harvey, and G. A. Hobart, "Potential Rhythms of the Cerebral Cortex During Sleep," *Science*, vol. 82, 1935, pp. 198–200.

[6] G. D. Dawson, "Cerebral Responses to Electrical Stimulation of Peripheral Nerve in Man," *J. Neurol. Neurosurg. Psychiatry*, vol. 10, 1947, pp. 134–140.

[7] G. D. Dawson, "A Summation Technique for the Detection of Small Evoked Potentials," *Electroencephalography and Clinical Neurophysiology*, vol. 6, 1954, pp. 65–84.

[8] G. Dietsch, "Fourier-analyse von Elektrenkephalogrammen des Menschen," *Pflüger's Arch. Ges. Physiol.*, vol. 230, 1932, pp. 106–112.

[9] E. Niedermayer, "Historical Aspects," in *Electroencephalography: Basic Principles, Clinical Applications and Related Fields*, 4th ed., Baltimore, MD: Williams & Wilkins, 1999, pp. 1–14.

[10] M. Nuwer, "Assesment of Digital EEG, Quantitative EEG, and EEG Brain Mapping: Report of the American Academy of Neurology and the American Clinical Neurophysiology Society," *Neurology*, vol. 49, 1997, pp. 277–292.

[11] P. J. Durka and K. J. Blinowska, "A Unified Time-Frequency Parametrization of EEG," *IEEE Engineering in Medicine and Biology Magazine*, vol. 20, no. 5, 2001, pp. 47–53.

[12] A. Rechtschaffen and A. Kales, (eds.), *A Manual of Standardized Terminology, Techniques and Scoring System for Sleep Stages in Human Subjects*, Number 204 in National Institutes of Health Publications, U.S. Government Printing Office, Washington, D.C., 1968.

[13] P. J. Durka, "Time-Frequency Analyses of EEG," Ph.D. thesis, Warsaw University, June 1996.

[14] J. Żygierewicz, et al., "High Resolution Study of Sleep Spindles," *Clinical Neurophysiology*, vol. 110, no. 12, 1999, pp. 2136–2147.

[15] P. J. Durka, et al., "High Resolution Parametric Description of Slow Wave Sleep," *Journal of Neuroscience Methods*, vol. 147, no. 1, 2005, pp. 15–21.

[16] E. Niedermayer and F. Lopes Da Silva, *Electroencephalography: Basic Principles, Clinical Applications and Related Fields*, 4th ed., Baltimore, MD: Williams & Wilkins, 1999.

[17] S. Mallat and Z. Zhang, "Matching Pursuit Software Package (mpp)," 1993, ftp://cs.nyu.edu/pub/wave/software/mpp.tar.Z.

[18] P. J. Durka, et al., "A Simple System for Detection of EEG Artifacts in Polysomnographic Recordings," *IEEE Transactions on Biomedical Engineering*, vol. 50, no. 4, 2003, pp. 526–528.

[19] D. J. Dijk, D. G. Beersma, and G. M. Bloem, "Sex Differences in the Sleep EEG of Young Adults: Visual Scoring and Spectral Analysis," *Sleep*, vol. 12, no. 6, 1989, pp. 500–507.

[20] H. Danker-Hopfe, et al., "Interrater Reliability Between Scorers from Eight European Sleep Laboratories in Subjects with Different Sleep Disorders," *Journal of Sleep Research*, vol. 13, no. 1, 2004, pp. 63–69.

[21] L. H. Larsen, et al., "A Note on the Night-to-Night Stability of Stages 3+4 Sleep in Healthy Older Adults: A Comparison of Visual and Spectral Evaluations of Stages 3+4 Sleep," *Sleep*, vol. 18, 1995, pp. 7–10.

[22] R. Armitage, et al., "Temporal Characteristics of Delta Activity During NREM Sleep in Depressed Outpatients and Healthy Adults: Group and Sex Effects," *Sleep*, vol. 23, no. 5, 2000, pp. 607–617.

[23] G. Bremer, J. R. Smith, and I. Karacan, "Automatic Detection of the K-Complex in Sleep Electroencephalograms," *IEEE Transactions on Biomedical Engineering*, vol. 17, 1970, pp. 314–323.

[24] P. J. Durka and K. J. Blinowska, "Analysis of EEG Transients by Means of Matching Pursuit," *Annals of Biomedical Engineering*, vol. 23, 1995, pp. 608–611.

[25] P. J. Durka, et al., "Adaptive Time-Frequency Parametrization in Pharmaco EEG," *Journal of Neuroscience Methods*, vol. 117, 2002, pp. 65–71.

[26] P. J. Durka, "Adaptive Time-Frequency Parametrization of Epileptic EEG Spikes," *Physical Review E*, vol. 69, no. 051914, 2004.

[27] M. Billiard, "The Standardized Sleep Manual, Love It or Leave It (guest editorial)," *Sleep Medicine Reviews*, vol. 4, no. 2, 2000, pp. 129–130.

[28] U. Malinowska, et al., "Micro- and Macrostructure of Sleep EEG," *IEEE BME Magazine*, vol. 25, 2006, pp. 26–31.

[29] M. Latka, et al., "Wavelet Analysis of Epileptic Spikes," *Physical Review E*, vol. 67, no. 052902, 2003.

Chapter 9

Epileptic Seizures

This chapter is devoted to the analysis of recordings of epileptic brain activity: from distinction between interictal spikes and their periodic series related to seizures, through delineation of stages of seizures in the time-frequency maps of signal energy density, to MP-derived statistical measures reflecting the increased complexity of the signal during seizures. Methodological issues addressed in this context include sensitivity of greedy algorithms to the periodicity of signal components and stopping criteria of MP decompositions.

In the previous section we analyzed single (separate) spikes and spike-wave complexes, which represent so-called interictal activity. The same structures, occurring within a periodic series (that is, equally spaced trains) are associated with epileptic seizures [1].

Epileptic seizures are abnormal, temporary manifestations of dramatically increased neuronal synchrony, either occurring regionally (partial seizures) or bilaterally (generalized seizures) in the brain [2]. However, all cerebral activity detectable by electroencephalography (i.e., EEG) is a reflection of synchronous neuronal activity.[1] Therefore, synchronous neuronal activity per se is not abnormal—at least below a certain threshold. In the following section we will address reflections of these processes in the EEG signal, in particular the transition from more or less randomly occurring spikes to their periodic trains.

1 Quoting from [3], "[...] enough evidence exists to state that the EEG on the scalp is mainly caused by synchronously occurring postsynaptic potentials." Large pools of neurons must act in synchrony to produce a signal strong enough to be measured at the scalp.

9.1 SERIES OF SPIKES

In decompositions from Figure 8.12, interictal spikes were parameterized by short, separate Gabor functions, represented as vertical blobs in the time-frequency plane. The same structures, occurring within a repeatable pattern (i.e., forming a periodic signal) can be represented as so-called Fourier series.[2] We encountered this kind of representation when discussing spectra in Chapter 3; for example, Figure 3.13 presents a harmonic approximation of a square wave. In general, the more a periodic waveform differs from a pure sine, the more harmonics are needed in a representation to explain its nonsinusoidal shape.

In the signal presented in Figure 9.1, spike-wave complexes occur at constant intervals, about three per second. The periodic part of the signal is represented as a series of structures elongated in time, located at harmonic frequencies starting around 3 Hz. However, the last three spikes are again represented as separate, transient structures. Although it may not be apparent from the signal itself, its MP representation suggests that these last three spikes belong to a period of loss of rhythmicity, which marks the end of the seizure. In Figure 9.2, about half of the spikes are represented as separate structures, and the other half as a harmonic series—this, in turn, may be related to the start of a seizure. The waves (i.e., wider structures accompanying spikes) are mostly represented as a harmonic series, namely the first two strong components around 3 Hz and 6 Hz.

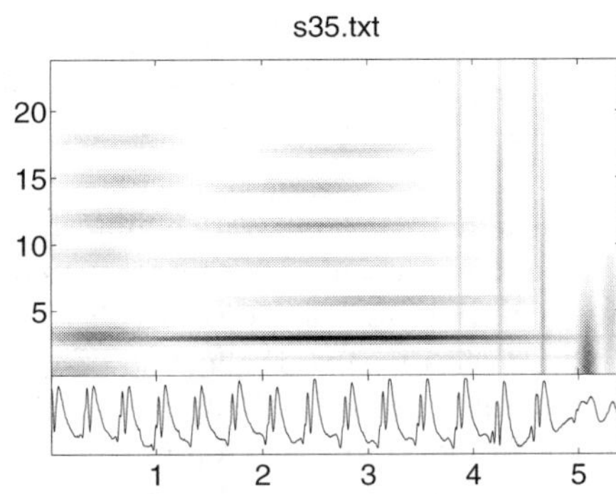

Figure 9.1 Periodic series of spike-wave complexes, represented (except for the last three) as rhythmic activity with base frequency around 3 Hz (horizontal structures from 0 to 3.5 seconds). (Signal courtesy of authors of [4].)

2 That is, as a sum of sines with frequencies being integer multiples of the basic frequency.

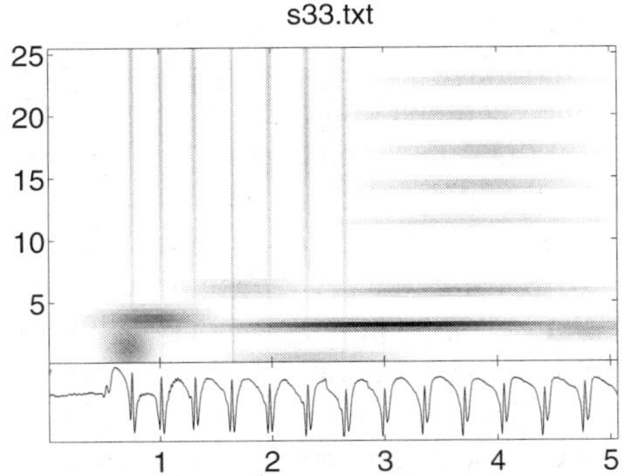

Figure 9.2 Another series of spike-wave complexes, where spikes before the third second are represented as separate structures, and after as rhythmic activity. Nonperiodicity of the first part, visible in the MP representation, can be also observed as minute deviations from the uniform distances between the maxima of the sharp peaks in the raw data. Like in Figure 9.1, first harmonic of the slow waves (2.9 Hz) is less sensitive to this effect. (Signal courtesy of authors of [4]. Reprinted figure with permission from [5]. © 2004 by the American Physical Society.)

Above a certain threshold of periodicity, trains of spikes are represented as Fourier series. Transitions to and from such strictly periodic states relate to different stages of seizures, described in Section 9.3. In the following section we will explain an intrinsic property of the MP algorithm, which clearly distinguishes strictly periodic components of the signal.

9.2 PERIODICITY AND GREEDY ALGORITHMS

As discussed in the first part of this book, basically any signal can be represented either in terms of its Fourier transform (i.e., weighted sum of sines) or as a sum of structures with better time localization, wider in the frequency domain. This choice is normally done a priori when selecting the method for analysis. Spectral methods (Chapter 3) correspond to variants of harmonic (i.e., Fourier) expansions. In the time-frequency methods (Chapter 4), the tradeoff between the time and frequency resolutions is regulated a priori by the parameters of the procedure (e.g., the width of the spectrogram window or chosen wavelet).

Adaptive approximations, and hence also the matching pursuit algorithm, are exceptions to this rule. Choice of the representation (that is, sharp spikes versus long sines in Figures 9.1 and 9.2) is an internal part of the procedure. In every step of the MP algorithm, this choice is based upon the content of the analyzed signal. Although this solution is elegant, convenient, and optimal, this optimality is only based upon a simple energetic criterion. We do not gain a direct insight into the system that generated the signal—mechanisms of generation of such abnormal rhythmic activity can be investigated by means of realistic computational models of neuronal networks (see [6]). However, in some cases, understanding the MP expansion allows us to infer—or at least hypothesize—about the nature of the underlying processes. For example, in the previous section we hypothesized about relations of the threshold between separate and harmonic representation of a series of spikes to the synchronization of brain activity, leading to epileptic seizures. Therefore, it is important to understand what an "optimal choice" actually means in the context of the matching pursuit decomposition.

The procedure governing this choice (i.e., the MP algorithm) was described in Section 5.3, and mathematical details are given in Section 13.5. Let us recall that matching pursuit breaks down the problem of finding a globally optimal representation into iterations. Briefly, *the algorithm chooses in each step the function that gives the largest product with the signal*—or more precisely the largest product with the residual (i.e., unexplained part of the signal left from the previous steps). This single-step optimization of the matching pursuit is often referred to as greedy, short-sighted, and—obviously—suboptimal strategy. It may be compared to a chess player looking only at gains in a single move. Just like a gambit in a chess game, choosing a function that explains less energy in a given step may lead in the following iterations to a better solution. For example, if all the spikes belonging to the series were parameterized separately by snugly fitting functions, the total residual error might have been smaller. However, in a single step, a sinusoidal function with humps of the oscillations fitting more or less approximately the whole periodic series of spikes may give a larger value of the product with the signal[3] than a narrow waveform, fitting perfectly a single spike.

Harmonic expansion is preferred only above a certain threshold of periodicity. This threshold defines a measure of periodicity of a series of spike-wave complexes, or any other repetitive structures. In the analysis of epileptic EEG spikes, this effect offers a clear distinction between a series of independent (or loosely related) events and rhythmic discharges. In the context of the detection algorithm, mentioned in Section 8.7, this feature provides a direct differentiation between separate (interictal) spikes and rhythmic discharges, related to seizures.

3 That is, it may explain more of the signal's energy. We mean here the product with the signal's residual $R^n x$, that is $\langle R^n x, g_{\gamma_n} \rangle$ from (13.11).

9.3 EVOLUTION OF SEIZURES

Observations from previous sections can be combined into a complete description of the evolution of seizures. Such a study was performed on intracranial EEG recordings (ICEEG) of mesial temporal onset partial seizures [7]. Whole epochs containing the seizures were subjected to MP decompositions. Although brain electrical activity in different stages of the seizures has clearly distinct properties, due to the adaptivity of the matching pursuit we can compute an efficient and high-resolution representation of the whole epoch at once, without prior subdivision into semi-stationary epochs.

Time-frequency estimates of signals' energy density, as those presented in Figures 9.3–9.5, were used in [7] as a basis for delineation of characteristic periods of the seizures. A general pattern of an organized rhythmic activity (ORA), characterized by one predominant periodic rhythm with monotonic decline of frequency, was found in the middle epoch of all the seizures. In Figure 9.4 it starts slightly after the fortieth second and ends near the one hundred fifth. First indications of abnormal activity are marked by a period of seizure initiation (INI), "[...] defined as the period before the persistent discernible change in the background could be identified. Various random interictal spikes or transients can be seen during this period, but no definite evolution occurs" [7]; in Figure 9.4 it occupies the first 30 seconds. Finally, periods preceeding and following the ORA—that is, transitional rhythmic activity (TRA, between INI and ORA) and intermittent bursting activity (IBA, after ORA)—were both characterized by a wide frequency spectrum of relatively high voltage. Due to the sensitivity of the MP algorithm to subtle transitions in frequency and phase, discussed in Section 8.5, we can clearly observe that these epochs comprise mostly short bursts of unsynchronized activity—contrary to the ORA period. These observations may be linked with hypotheses, which relate the synchronization and desynchronization, starting and terminating seizures, with periodicity observed in the series of spikes (discussed in the previous section).

On the purely methodological side, we observe that the harmonics of changing frequency, present in Figure 9.4 between 50 and 105 seconds, are represented by series of Gabor functions. This is due to the fact that in the Gabor dictionary only structures of constant frequency are available. This may be viewed as a limitation of the method; in theory, MP algorithm can be implemented with a dictionary made of more or less any set of functions.[4] However, adding new degrees of freedom would

4 The only requirement for the convergence of MP is that these functions suffice to explain any signal (i.e., form a dense set).

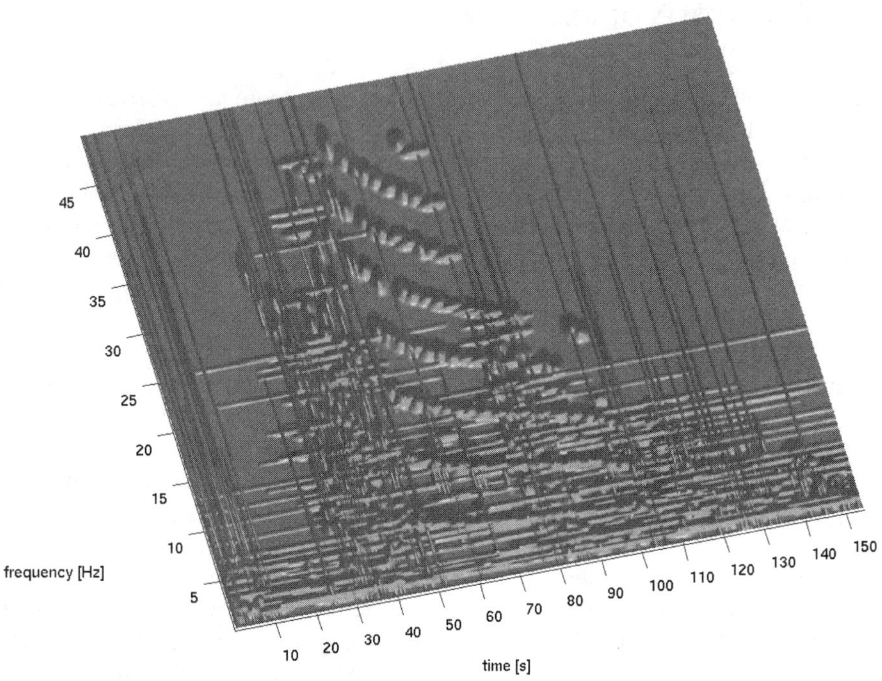

Figure 9.3 Three-dimensional representation of the time-frequency energy density, calculated from MP decomposition of an intracranial recording (ICEEG) of an epileptic seizure. The same distribution is presented in Figure 9.4 in two dimensions, together with the decomposed ICEEG. Both pictures illustrate different dynamical states, identified in [7]. Near the thirtieth second, the period of seizure initiation (INI) transforms into transitional rhythmic activity (TRA). Slightly after the fortieth second, the organized rhythmic activity (ORA)—with eight clearly visible harmonics of the main, decreasing frequency—becomes dominant, to dissolve into intermittent bursting activity (IBA) near the one hundred fifth second. (ICEEG recording courtesy of Professor P. J. Franaszczuk and Professor G. K. Bergey; interpretation after [7].)

significantly complicate both the decomposition and the intepretation of results (see also Sections 7.4 and 13.10).

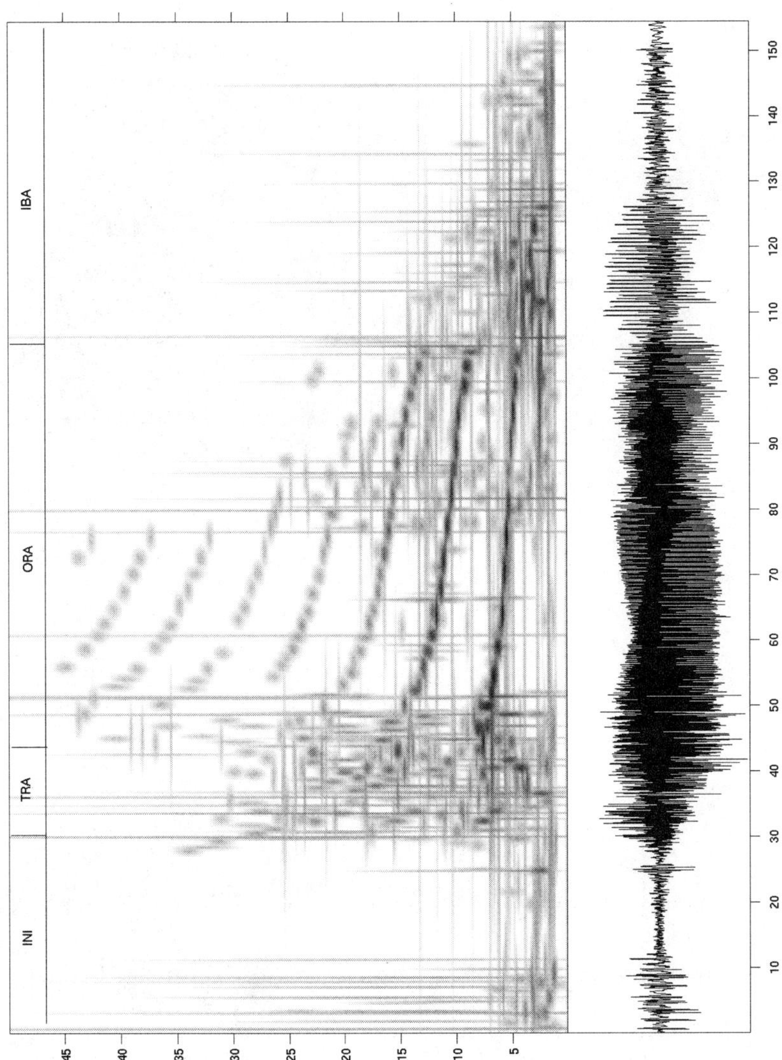

Figure 9.4 Two-dimensional representation of energy density of the intracranial recording (ICEEG) from Figure 9.3. Horizontal axis—time [s], vertical (on the time-frequency plot) [Hz]. (ICEEG recording courtesy of Professor P. J. Franaszczuk and Professor G. K. Bergey; interpretation after [7].)

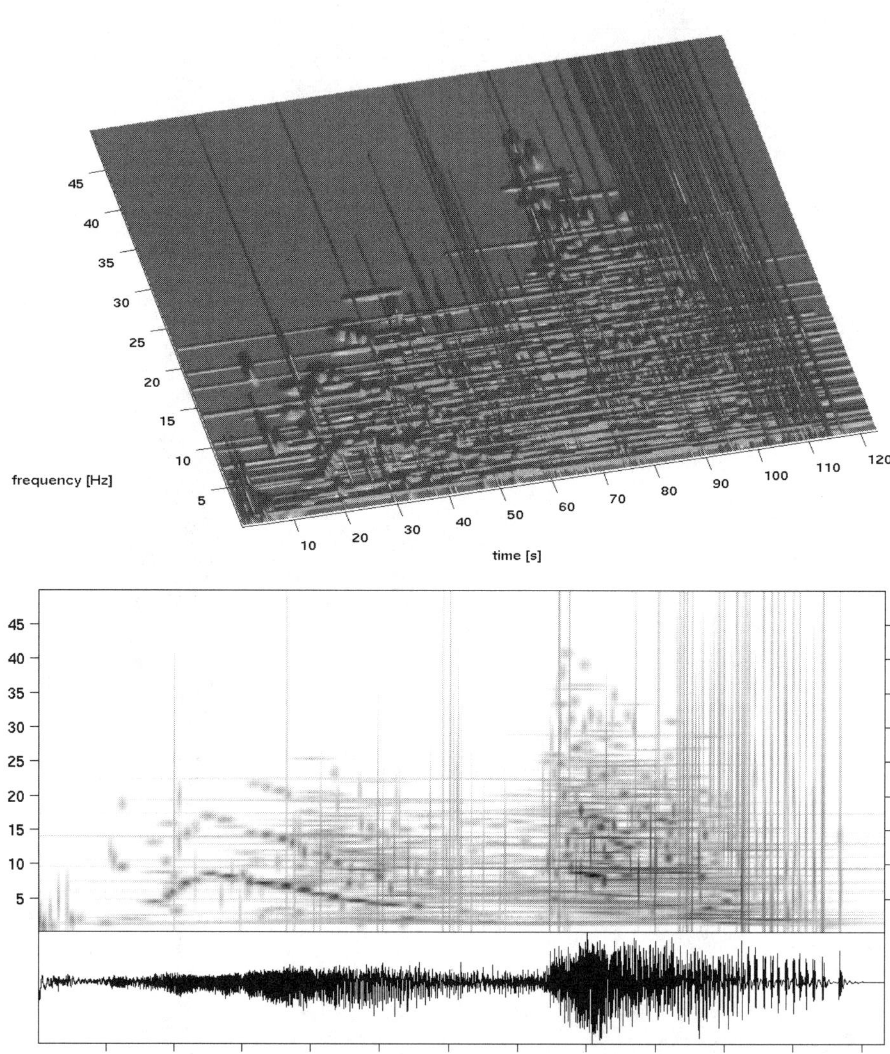

Figure 9.5 ICEEG recording of another seizure and MP-derived distributions of energy as in Figures 9.3 and 9.4. (ICEEG recording courtesy of Professor P. J. Franaszczuk and Professor G. K. Bergey.)

9.4 GABOR ATOM DENSITY

Analysis of ICEEG recorded during epileptic seizures, presented in the previous section, revealed characteristic periods occurring in most of the recordings. They were clearly visible in the time-frequency estimates of signals' energy density, but their delineation required visual inspection of these maps. Such methods inherit some of the drawbacks of visual analysis (see Section 8.3) and are not suitable for an automated detection of seizures or online monitoring. On the other hand, if the characteristic periods can be reliably delineated in the time-frequency maps, then the relevant information must be contained also in the MP decomposition underlying their construction. This has motivated the authors of [8] to develop an objective statistical measure, which would describe the complexity of the signal perceived in the time-frequency maps. It was based upon the observation that increased complexity of the signal in the seizure periods relates to a higher number of time-frequency atoms, used by the MP algorithm to explain the signal in a given time epoch. We can observe this effect in Figure 9.6, where centers of atoms from the MP decompositions from Figures 9.3 and 9.4 are marked by crosses in the time-frequency plane.

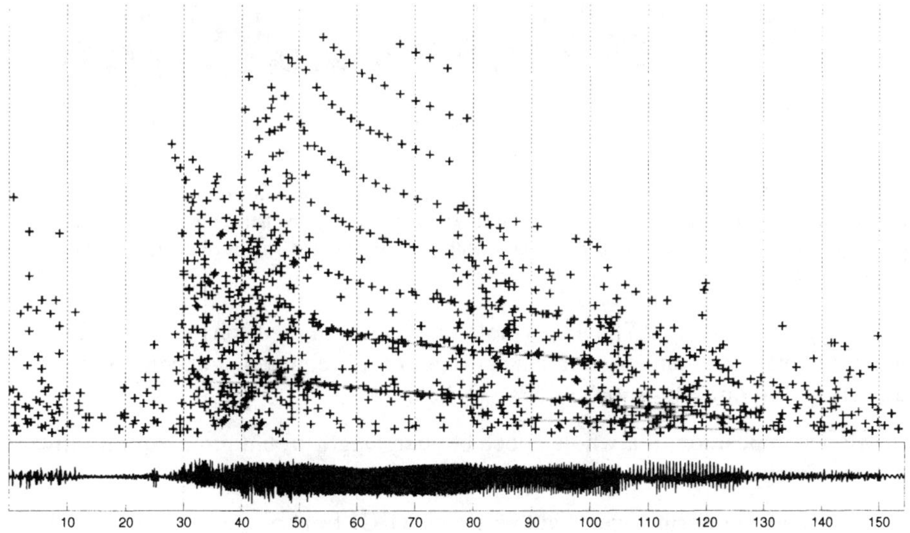

Figure 9.6 Representation from Figure 9.4, with centers of atoms marked by the crosses. Vertical lines symbolize possible division into subepochs.

A measure of this effect was termed Gabor atom density (GAD) [8]. GAD is calculated as the number of atoms in an MP decomposition per unit of time, but it actually corresponds to the density of atoms in the time-frequency plane: for sampling frequency f_s, the frequency axis goes from 0 to $f_s/2$, so the volume of a slice encompassing the whole frequency will be proportional to the time length of the slice. Plate 4 presents the time course of GAD superimposed on the time-frequency representation calculated for a 10-minute ICEEG recording containing a seizure with pre- and postictal epochs. We observe that the value of GAD in preictal and postictal periods fluctuates slightly above 0.1 (scale on the right), while in the ictal period it displays values between 0.25 and 0.4. Suitability of this measure for online monitoring and automated seizure detection is represented in Figure 9.7, which gives the time course of GAD over a whole day plus a 90-minute period comprising a seizure (marked by an arrow).

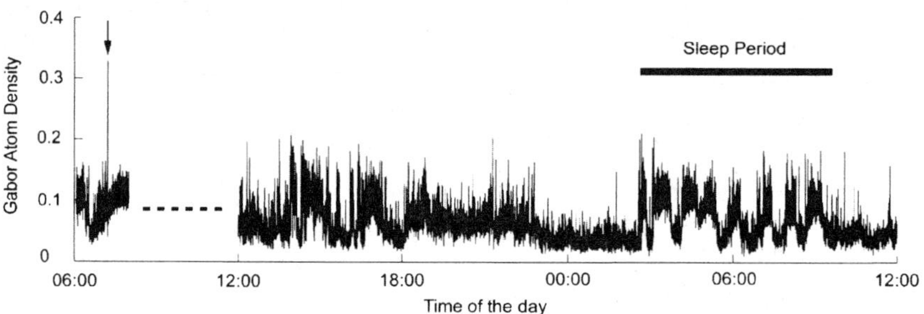

Figure 9.7 GAD time course over a 90-minute period with a 1-minute seizure and a consecutive 24-hour seizure-free period. The seizure is indicated by the arrow. The horizontal black bar indicates the sleep period. (Reprinted from [8], © 2003, with permission from The International Federation of Clinical Neurophysiology.)

Although Figure 9.7 gives a whole-day course of GAD changes, it cannot be estimated from the number of atoms per unit of time, counted in decompositions of the whole 24-hour-long epoch of ICEEG, because:

1. MP decomposition of a whole epoch of such length would require prohibitively large computing resources.
2. For online monitoring, we need to estimate GAD from possibly short epochs.

Therefore, we have to compare the numbers of atoms counted in separate MP decompositions of a priori chosen subepochs. For a reliable realization of this task we have to take into account the criterion applied for stopping the MP decomposition, which effectively regulates the number of atoms in the expansion. This issue has been only briefly mentioned in Section 7.2; stopping criteria of MP algorithm will be formally discussed in Section 13.7.

The simplest criterion, relatively robust in routine applications, fixes a priori the number of algorithm iterations, regardless of the content of the analyzed signal. Obviously, its application here would result in a flat time course of GAD. Another simple criterion can be based upon the percentage of the signal's energy, explained by the MP expansion. But its actual performace may fluctuate wildly. For example, while 95%–98% of energy in an EEG epoch may normally contain most of the relevant structures, it is not impossible that one strong structure, such as low frequency artifact, saturates 90% of the signal's energy, terminating the decomposition well before addressing the relevant content.

Coherence criterion proposed in [9] relies on the relative amount of energy, explained in every iteration. Its value is calculated as the ratio of the energy of the atom, added in a given iteration, to the energy of the residual left from the previous one. Expected value of this criterion can be estimated for the case of decomposing a white noise (of a length equal to the length of the analyzed signal). If we reach this value during decomposition of the signal, it may indicate that we reached a point where in the residual there are no more structures coherent with the signal, and further iterations will not contribute much information. However, this criterion is based upon the energy of the residuals, and it may exhibit variable performance for signals of different properties.

Ultimately we are looking for a criterion that, when applied to the decomposition of subepochs, would result in relative counts of atoms similar[5] to the numbers counted within the corresponding slices of the decomposition of the whole epoch.

This idea is visualized in Figure 9.6, where vertical lines divide the signal into 10-second example subepochs and its time-frequency representation into corresponding slices. Let us contemplate this figure for a while. No matter what criterion was used for stopping the underlying MP decomposition, we can find the energy of the last atom added in the last iteration; let's denote it E_{last}. We may ensure that decompositions of the subepochs are stopped exactly after reaching the same value of the signal's energy explained by the last atom. Then—apart from the unavoidable

5 There are some intrinsic differences between the decomposition of the whole epoch calculated at once and separate decompositions of its subepochs. We cannot compensate for a possible presence of structures longer than subepochs and, especially, for the increased influence of border effects in subepoch decompositions. Relative influence of border conditions depends on the size of the analyzed signal, so in decompositions of subepochs of constant length, this effect can be more or less constant.

differences resulting from the border conditions in shorter subepochs—counts of atoms from the decompositions of subepochs, stopped after reaching E_{last}, would correspond to the number of atoms counted within the corresponding time slices of decomposition of the whole epoch.

This stopping criterion, based upon the energy of the last added atom, can be seen as the achieved energy resolution of the decomposition, hence it was termed "energy resolution criterion" or "energy threshold criterion" [8]. This criterion was also proposed in [10] (and proved in [11]) as leading to an expansion optimal in the rate/distortion sense in a similar problem involving MP decompositions of subparts of images in video coding. Performance of GAD estimates based upon both the coherence and energy resolution criteria was evaluated in [8]. After few more years of experience with GAD, the authors switched completely to the energy resolution criterion (Christophe C. Jouny, personal communication, 2006).

Finally, we can explain (after [8]) how the GAD time courses—presented in Plate 4 and Figure 9.7—were actually calculated. The signal, subsampled to 100 Hz, was divided into 10.24-second long epochs with a 200-point (2 seconds) shift, resulting in a 2-second time resolution.[6] These epochs were subjected to MP decomposition into a large number of waveforms. Computing the values of GAD—using the energy resolution criterion—relies on a threshold (i.e., maximum energy of the last atom in decomposition). The value of this threshold was not known a priori: it was optimized to enhance the differences in GAD between selected periods of seizures and the background level.

From the first seizure of each patient, the difference was calculated between the GAD maximum level during the ictal period and the mean GAD level over 200 seconds before the seizure onset. This optimization did not require additional calculations, since the energy thresholds can be applied as restrictions on the previously calculated decompositions, stored on disk (if we perform these decompositions with sufficiently large setting for the number of waveforms).

Clinical interpretation of results can be found in [8]. Stopping criteria of the MP algorithm are further discussed in Section 13.7.

6 This particular length of the epoch—1,024 points—was chosen as the power of 2 closest to 1,000 points (i.e., 10 seconds), since epoch lengths equal to powers of 2 are preferable for the FFT routines inside the software package (mpp) by Mallat and Zhang [12], used in this study for the MP decompositions.

References

[1] F. A. Gibbs and H. Davis, "Changes in the Human Electroencephalogram Associated with Loss of Consciousness," *Am. J. Physiol*, vol. 113, 1935, pp. 49–50.

[2] G. K. Bergey and P. J. Franaszczuk, "Epileptic Seizures Are Characterized by Changing Signal Complexity," *Clinical Neurophysiology*, vol. 112, 2001, pp. 241–249.

[3] E. Niedermayer and F. Lopes Da Silva, *Electroencephalography: Basic Principles, Clinical Applications and Related Fields*, 4th ed., Baltimore, MD: Williams & Wilkins, 1999.

[4] M. Latka, et al., "Wavelet Analysis of Epileptic Spikes," *Physical Review E*, vol. 67, no. 052902, 2003.

[5] P. J. Durka, "Adaptive Time-Frequency Parametrization of Epileptic EEG Spikes," *Physical Review E*, vol. 69, no. 051914, 2004.

[6] M. de Curtis and G. Avanzini, "Interictal Spikes in Focal Epileptogenesis," *Progress in Neurobiology*, vol. 63, 2001, pp. 541–567.

[7] P. J. Franaszczuk, et al., "Time-Frequency Analysis Using the Matching Pursuit Algorithm Applied to Seizures Originating from the Mesial Temporal Lobe," *Electroencephalography and Clinical Neurophysiology*, vol. 106, 1998, pp. 513–521.

[8] C. C. Jouny, P. J. Franaszczuk, and G. K. Bergey, "Characterization of Epileptic Seizure Dynamics Using Gabor Atom Density," *Clinical Neurophysiology*, vol. 114, 2003, pp. 426–437.

[9] S. Mallat and Z. Zhang, "Matching Pursuit with Time-Frequency Dictionaries," *IEEE Transactions on Signal Processing*, vol. 41, December 1993, pp. 3397–3415.

[10] R. Neff and A. Zakhor, "Modulus Quantization for Matching Pursuit Video Coding," *IEEE Transactions on Circuits and Systems for Video Technology*, vol. 10, no. 6, January 2000, pp. 13–26.

[11] C. de Vleeschouwer and A. Zakhor, "In-Loop Atom Modulus Quantization for Matching Pursuit and Its Application to Video Coding," *IEEE Transactions on Image Processing*, vol. 12, no. 10, October 2003, pp. 1226–1242.

[12] S. Mallat and Z. Zhang, "Matching Pursuit Software Package (mpp)," 1993, ftp://cs.nyu.edu/pub/wave/software/mpp.tar.Z.

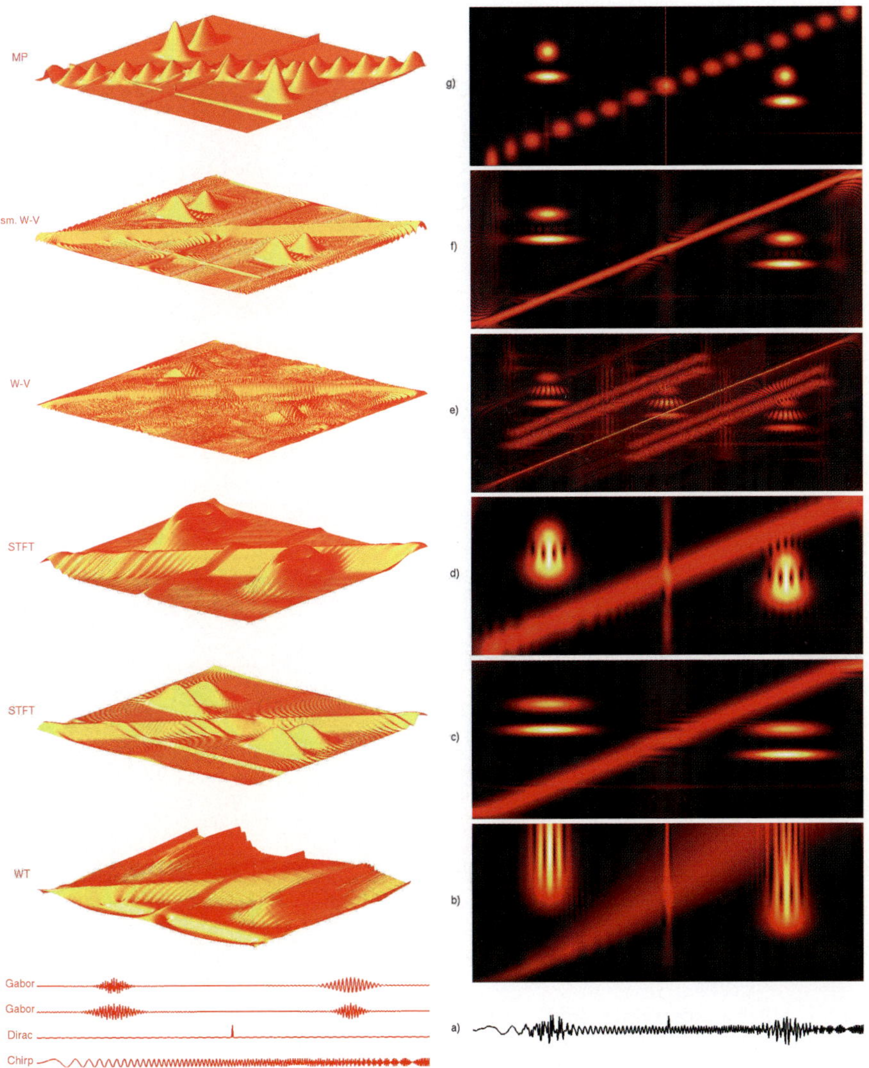

Plate 1: Estimates of time-frequency energy density of a simulated signal (a), containing four Gabor functions, Dirac's delta, and chirp (bottom left, red). (b) Wavelet transform. (c), (d) Spectrograms with different window lengths. (e) Wigner-Ville transform. (f) Smoothed W-V with kernel adjusted for optimal representation of this signal. (g) Matching pursuit. For discussion, see Section 6.2.

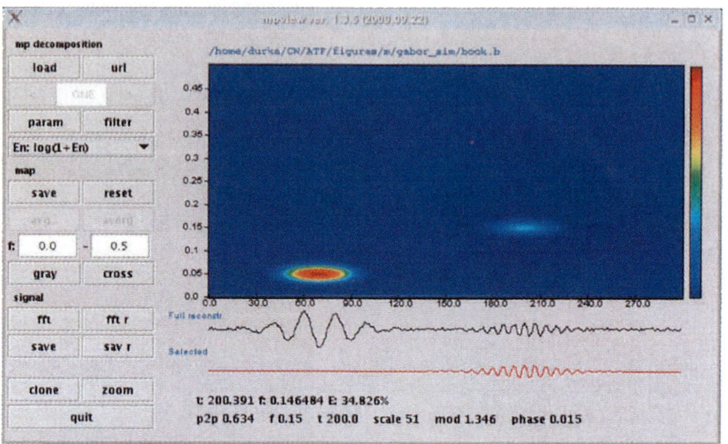

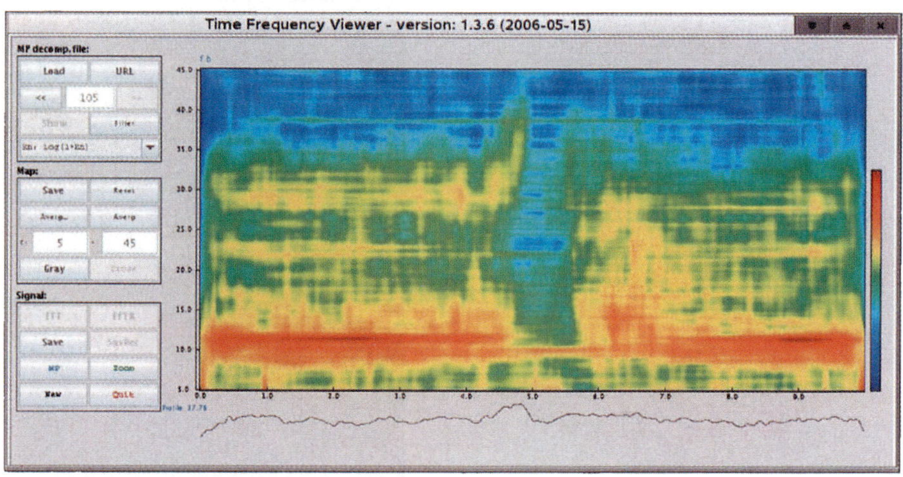

Plate 2: MPview, an interactive program for exploring results of MP decompositions. Upper screenshot: simulated signal from Section 5.3, the black trace below the time-frequency map gives reconstruction of the signal. The red trace presents reconstruction of functions chosen by clicking their time-frequency centers. Numbers relate to the current position of the cursor above the time-frequency map (time, frequency, and energy density) and the parameters of the nearest time-frequency atom. Lower panel: average energy density for data from Section 10.2, presented also in Plate 5; the black trace gives energy versus time. Program written in Java by D. Ircha (dobi@message.pl), available from http://eeg.pl/mp.

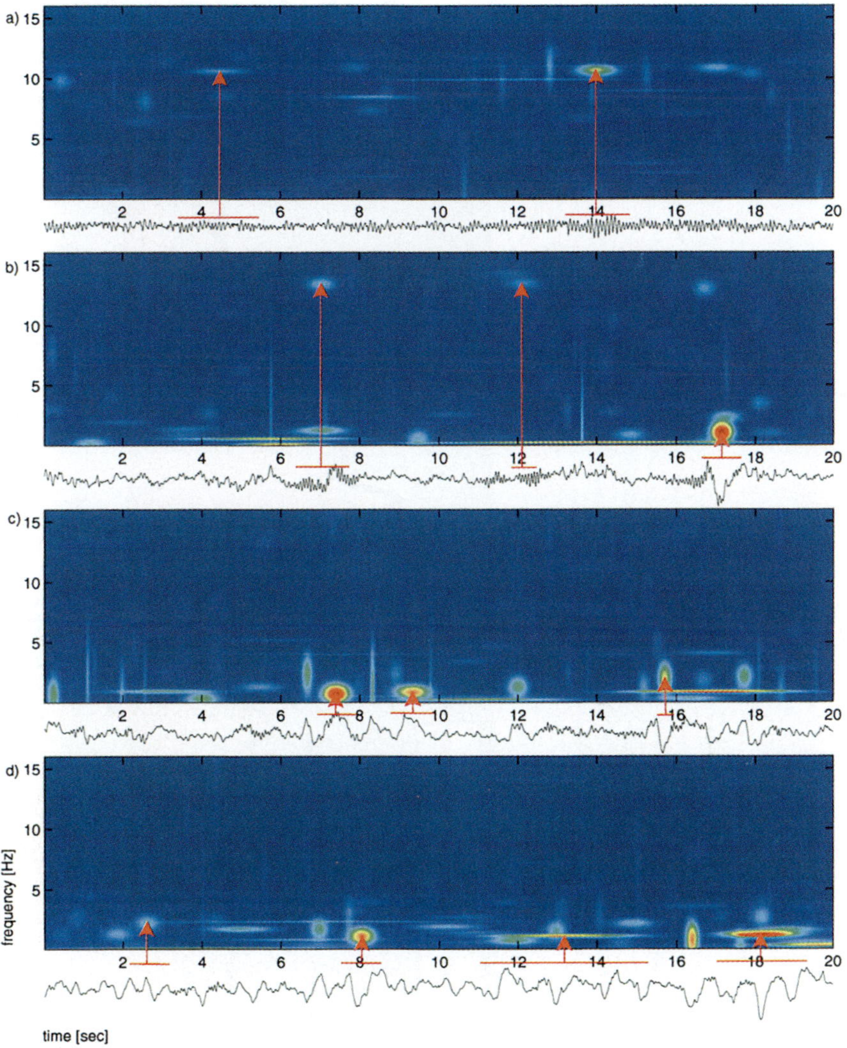

Plate 3: Time-frequency maps of energy derived from MP decompositions of 20-second epochs of EEG in different behavioral states. Energy scale from blue (zero) to red (max). Red arrows connect relevant EEG structures with the corresponding blobs in the time-frequency plane. (a) Wake: marked alpha, (b) sleep stage 2: marked two sleep spindles and K-complex, (c) and (d) sleep stages 3 and 4, respectively, marked slow waves. (*From:* [28] in Chapter 8. © 2006 IEEE. Reprinted with permission.)

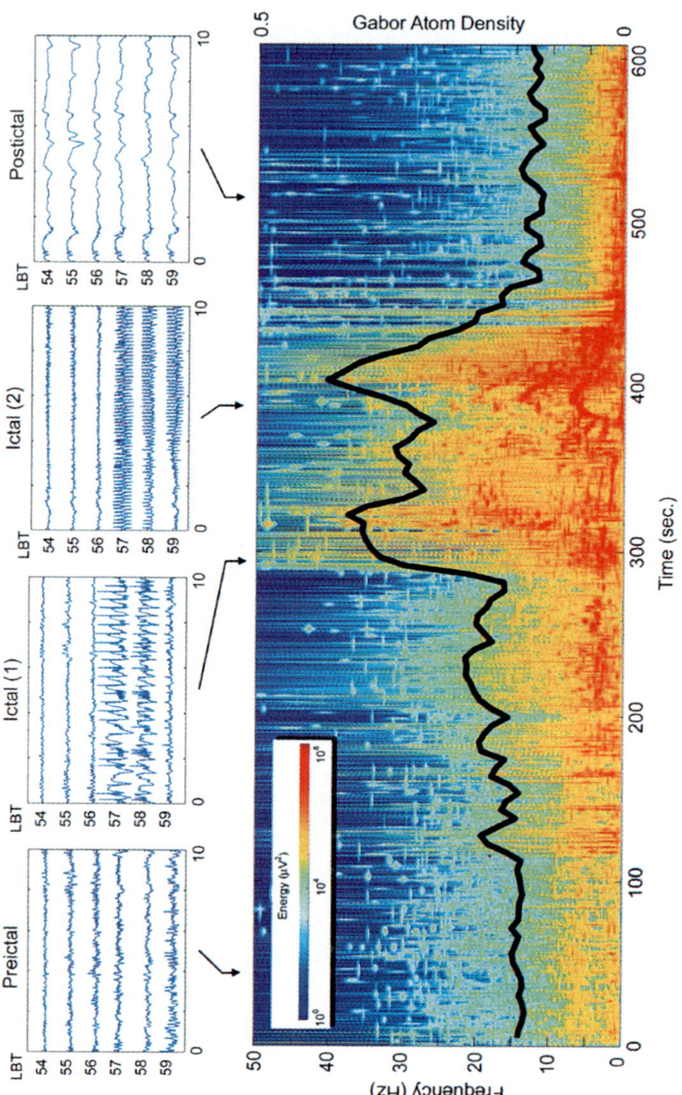

Plate 4: Time course of GAD superimposed on the corresponding time-frequency map. (Reprinted from [8] in Chapter 9, © 2003, with permission from The International Federation of Clinical Neurophysiology.)

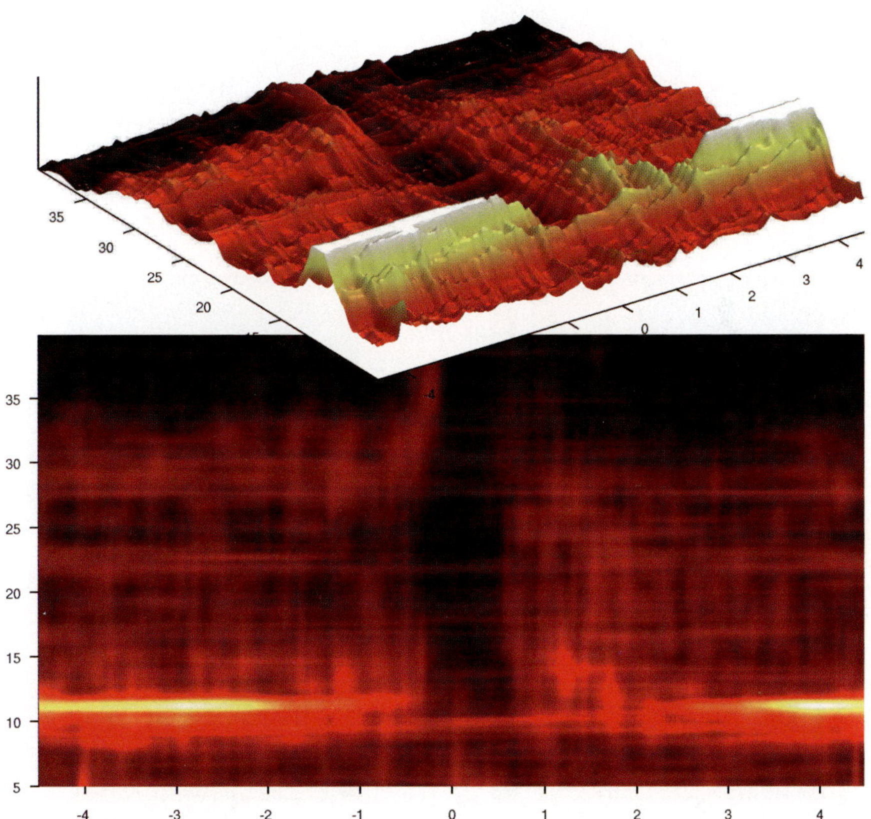

Plate 5: Average time-frequency energy density calculated from the matching pursuit expansion for the data from Figure 10.2. Horizontal scale represents seconds relative to the finger movement; vertical scale represents frequency (Hz). Top—the same in three dimensions, but energy of the alpha band is cut off in 50% of the height to show weaker high-frequency structures. (From [5] in Chapter 10, reprinted with permission. © 2001 by Springer.)

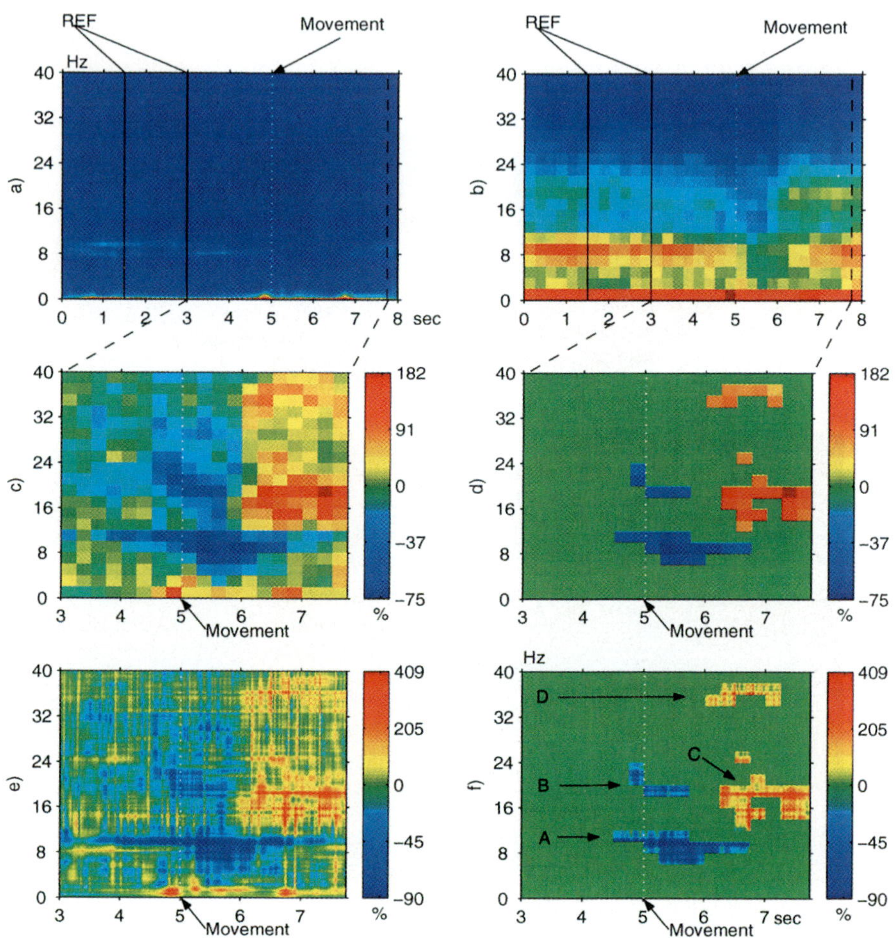

Plate 6: (a) Average time-frequency energy density, calculated from MP decomposition of EEG from a standard fingertapping experiment (movement onset in the fifth second). (b) Energy from (a) integrated in resels 0.25 seconds×2 Hz. (c) Average values of ERD/ERS. (d) Regions from (c) indicated as statistically different from the reference epoch by pseudo-t bootstrap procedure corrected by a 5% FDR. (e) High-resolution map of ERD/ERS calculated from (a). (f) High-resolution ERD/ERS in statistically significant regions from (d): A—μ desynchronization, B—desynchronization of the μ harmonic, C—post-movement β synchronization, D—harmonic of β. (From [10] in Chapter 10. © 2004 IEEE. Reprinted with permission.)

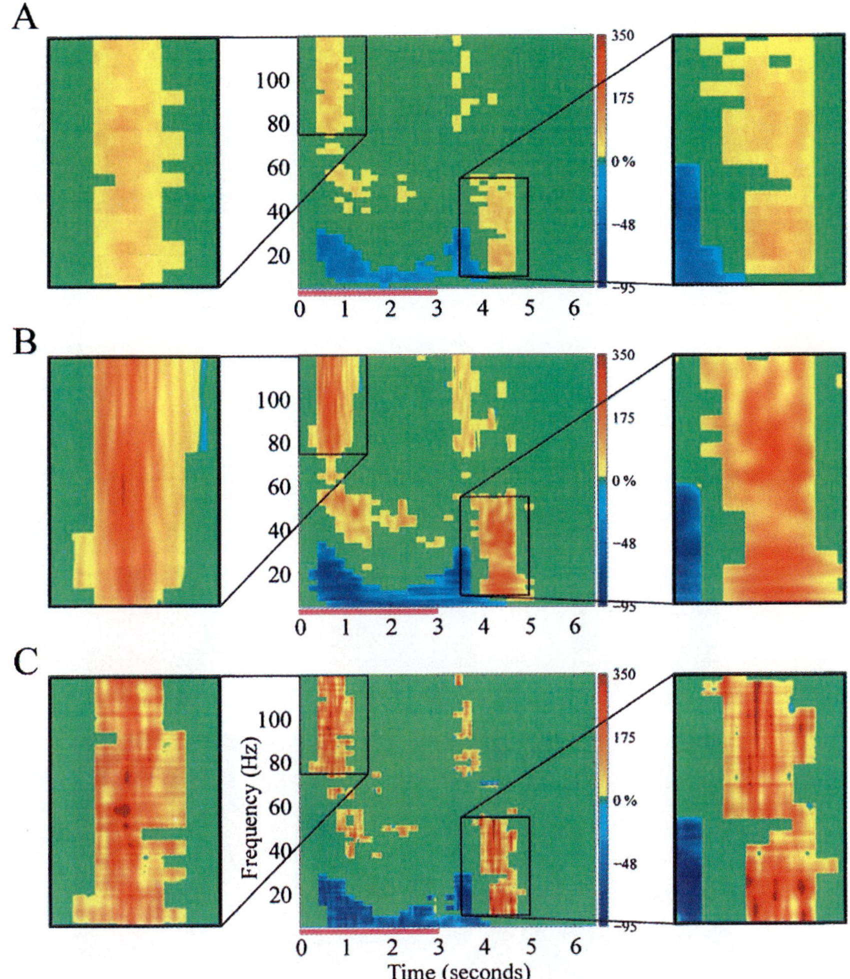

Plate 7: Time-frequency maps of significant ERD/ERS in ECoG data from [22,23] in Chapter 10, calculated as presented in Plate 6. Left column—enlarged fragment of maps showing high gamma (>75 Hz) ERS; right column—expanded ERS in lower frequencies (<30 Hz); middle column shows the original maps. Horizontal magenta bar on the time axis indicates the duration of the visual cue for muscle contraction. Rows: A—spectrogram, B—scalogram, C—MP estimates of energy density. (Reprinted from [9] in Chapter 10, © 2005, with permission from Elsevier.)

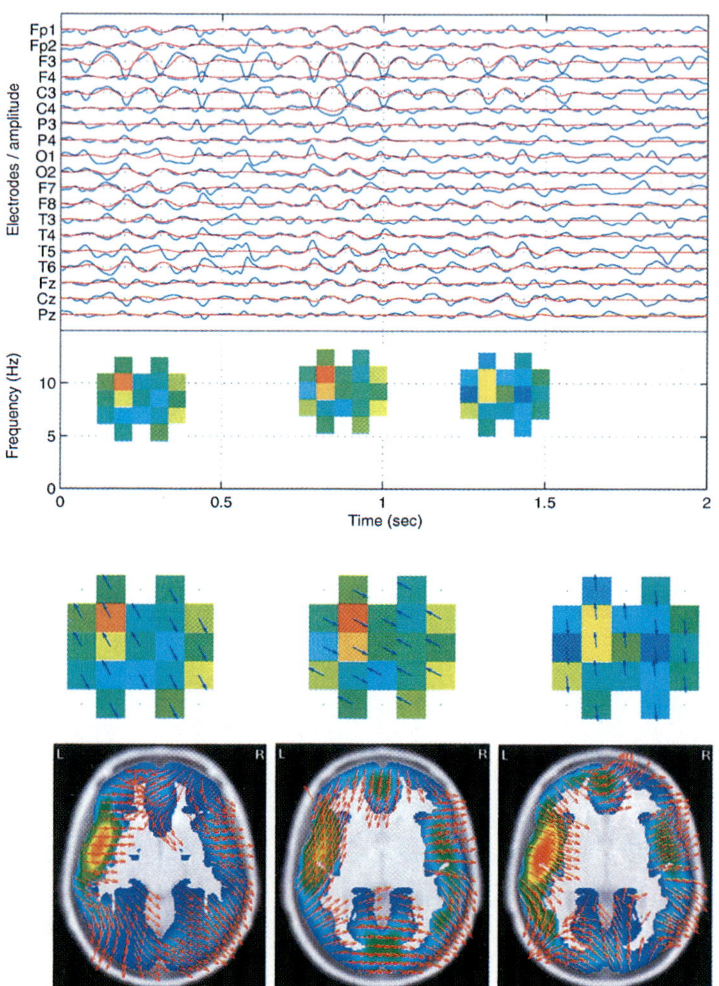

Plate 8: Upper plot—2 seconds of EEG (blue trace, data from [22] in Section 12) and reconstructions (red) of selected Gabor atoms. Distributions of their amplitudes on electrodes (10–20 system as in Table 8.2, front of the head upwards) are displayed below in corresponding time-frequency positions. Middle row—the same topographies with phases marked by arrows. Lower row—horizontal slices from distributed EEG inverse solution (LORETA) computed from each of these topographies, with colors indicating primary current densities estimated in each voxel, and arrows marking their directions. Recomputed by A. Matysiak using algorithm MMP1 (Section 13.12).

Chapter 10

Event-Related Desynchronization and Synchronization

This chapter presents high-resolution time-frequency maps of event-related desynchronization (ERD) and synchronization (ERS) of EEG and ECoG, including complete framework for estimation of their significance. Adaptivity of MP estimates is compared to the spectrogram and scalogram.

Desynchronization of brains' electrical activity in response to external stimuli was first reported by Adolf Beck (Figure 10.1) in 1890. Quoting [1]:

> In his very first experiment (on a rabbit) Beck found an oscillating potential difference between two electrodes placed on the occipital cortex. The fluctuations ceased when he uncovered the animal's eyes and lit a magnesium flare, and they also ceased with stimulation of the hind leg. [...] Thus to Caton's discoveries, Beck had added yet another—that of desynchronization of cortical activity following afferent stimulation. This phenomenon, confirmed later by many, remained an empirical observation for almost sixty years, until the elucidation of the desynchronizing action on cortical potentials of the ascending reticular system.

Beck was reading the potential changes from the exposed rabbit's cortex by observing the galvanometer connected directly to the electrodes, without an amplifier. Later, these findings were more precisely expressed in terms of blocking of the alpha band rhythms by Hans Berger [2], on some of the first photographic records of human EEG.

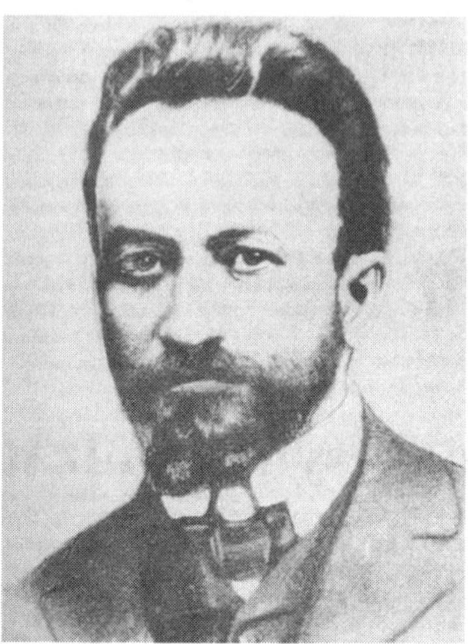

Figure 10.1 Adolf Beck (1863–1942), who discovered event-related EEG desynchronization. He was also the first to report the discovery of EEG—which he did independent of Caton's earlier work from 1875—in a widely read physiological journal [3].

10.1 CONVENTIONAL ERD/ERS QUANTIFICATION

Half a century later, quantitative measures of event-related desynchronization and synchronization (ERD and ERS) were introduced as time courses of the average changes of energy, relative to a reference epoch [4]. The classical method of quantification of ERD/ERS consists of time averaging the squared values of the samples of single trials, band-pass filtered in a priori selected bands. In the following we quote from [5] the classical procedure of ERD/ERS quantification using the dataset of a subject who participated in several studies [6–8]:

> [...] Movement-reactive frequency components were detected by comparing power spectral densities in the reference interval—chosen between 4.5 and 3.5 seconds before the movement onset—and in a 1-second period around the movement (–0.5 to +0.5 s). Frequency bands, showing significant differences between the reference interval and the activity interval, were chosen for ERD/ERS computations. The EEG was digitally band pass filtered in the selected bands (alpha band 10–12 Hz; beta band 14–18 Hz; gamma band 36–40 Hz) and power values were computed by squaring the samples and averaging these power samples across trials. To reduce the number of power values, 16

consecutive samples were averaged producing an 8 Hz sampling rate in the resulting power time series (original signal was sampled 128 Hz). Absolute band power was converted to percentage power using the reference interval as 100%. By convention, an ERD corresponds to power decrease and an ERS to a power increase.

Figure 10.2 depicts the ERD/ERS time courses for the following bands: 10–12, 14–18, and 36–40 Hz. The alpha band (mu) desynchronization (10–12 Hz) starts 2.5 seconds before movement-onset, reaches maximal desynchronization shortly after movement-onset, and recovers to baseline level within a few seconds. The central beta activity (14–18 Hz), in contrast, displays a short-lasting ERD during initiation of movement followed by a synchronization (ERS) with a maximum after the movement execution. It is of interest that the beta ERS occurs while the mu rhythm still shows a desynchronization. The 40-Hz oscillations (36–40 Hz) reveal a sharp power increase shortly before movement-onset.

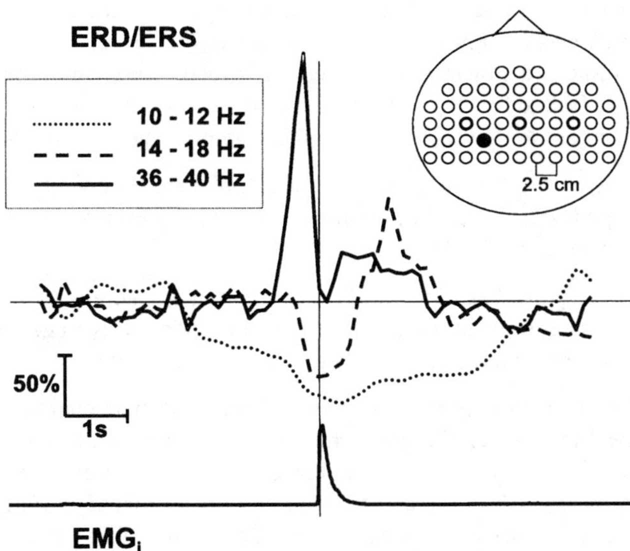

Figure 10.2 ERD/ERS in three bands: 10–12 Hz (α), 14–18 Hz (β), 36–40 Hz (γ). Insert: electrode positions C3, Cz, and C4 from the 10-20 system marked by thicker circles. Presented curves were computed for the electrode marked by the filled circle. (From [5], reprinted with permission. © 2001 by Springer.)

10.2 A COMPLETE TIME-FREQUENCY PICTURE

Classical ERD/ERS curves, described in the previous section, are naturally embedded in the time-frequency plane. A complete picture of mean event-related changes of energy density can be obtained as a sum of properly aligned estimates, computed for single trials. Such a sum will enhance event-related phenomena of similar time-frequency signatures—that is, occurring in the same time-frequency regions, as related to the trigger—regardless of their phase relations. This fact is hereby stressed in contrast to the standard averaging of the evoked potentials in time domain (see Figure 8.1), which enhances only the phase-locked components. Plate 5 presents such a distribution, calculated from the same EEG data as the ERD/ERS curves presented in the previous section. This picture was produced as follows:

1. Single EEG trials—the same as used for Figure 10.2—were subjected to the MP decomposition,[1] as described in Section 5.3 or (13.7) from Section 13.5. From the functions fitted to the signal, those corresponding to structures of duration below 0.125 seconds were excluded from the expansion. This can be understood as a kind of nonlinear denoising and corresponds to the time smoothing of curves from Figure 10.2 by a 16-point window. A parallel procedure (exclusion of structures longer than 4 seconds) was used to remove sharp frequency artifacts.
2. For each trial, a time-frequency map of the signal's energy density was calculated from the expansion obtained in the previous step, as described in Section 5.4 or (13.23) from Section 13.10.
3. Finally, all the time-frequency maps constructed for single trials—aligned in time relative to the event—were added, to produce an average (across trials) distribution of the signal's energy in the time-frequency plane.

Plate 5 presents this distribution in two dimensions, with energy density coded in a color scale. In the upper plot, the same distribution is presented as a 3-D surface, with energy corresponding to the height. Presentation of a complete, high resolution picture of energy changes eliminates the trial-and-error procedure of delineating the reactive frequency bands and provides a detailed insight into the time-frequency microstructure of the underlying processes.

How does the picture from Plate 5 relate to the classical ERD/ERS curves presented in Figure 10.2? As already mentioned, these curves are naturally embedded in the time-frequency plane. The classical procedure of estimating average signal

1 This book is about matching pursuit, so we use this estimate as the default. Other estimates of time-frequency energy density, mentioned in Part I, will be discussed in this context in Section 10.4.

energy in selected frequency bands relates to the integration of the power density from Plate 5 in these bands. Slices from this energy distribution, corresponding to the bands chosen in Figure 10.2, are presented in Figure 10.3. Classical procedure used for calculating ERD/ERS curves in these bands corresponds to integration of these slices along the frequency dimension. To obtain the numerical values of ERD/ERS, we divide the values obtained from integration by the average value of energy in this band, calculated for the reference period—in this experiment, they were chosen from 4.5 to 3.5 seconds before the movement.

This procedure gives a different estimate of the same ERD/ERS curves; high resolution of the MP-based method results in an increased selectivity of the energy estimate and hence also increased sensitivity to the ERD/ERS. For example, by comparing Figures 10.2 and 10.3, we find that the maximum ERS in the gamma band, reaching 200% in the classical estimates from Figure 10.2, is an order of magnitude stronger when calculated in exactly the same way from the selective MP estimate of energy density. Further possibility of enhancing the selectivity of matching pursuit estimates of energy of structures, originating in given frequency bands, will be discussed in Section 11.1.

10.3 ERD/ERS IN THE TIME-FREQUENCY PLANE

As a natural continuation of these considerations, we may calculate a time-frequency map of ERD/ERS by dividing the values displayed in Plate 5 by the average energy density in the reference epoch, calculated for each frequency separately. This also requires a choice of the frequency resolution; for spectrogram it will relate to the natural resolution of Fourier transform related to the chosen length of the analysis window, while for quadratic time-frequency distributions it will be chosen more or less arbitrarily.

However, such a ratio of two stochastic variables may exhibit even higher variance than the original energy distributions, so we may expect large fluctuations in the ERD/ERS time-frequency maps. Therefore, before drawing any conclusions from such maps, we need to account for the stochastic character of the signal and the occurrence of EEG structures unrelated to the event, which may produce an accidental increase or decrease of average energy density in relation to the reference epoch. Purely statistical issues, related to the significance of ERD/ERS in the time-frequency plane, are outside the main scope of this book, so the mathematical treatment of this problem is presented in Chapter 15.

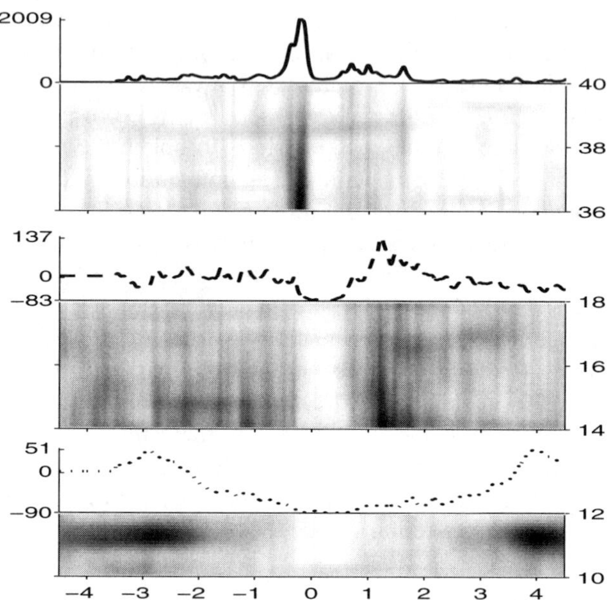

Figure 10.3 Slices from the time-frequency distribution presented in Plate 5, corresponding to the fixed bands chosen for the presentation in Figure 10.2. Curves above each plot are frequency integrals of the corresponding distributions (below each curve). Vertical axes on their left sides indicate percent of change, relative to energy integrated between 3.5 and 4.5 seconds before the movement in given band. (From [5], reprinted with permission. © 2001 by Springer.)

In brief, a complete procedure, leading to the display of statistically significant ERD/ERS in the time-frequency plane, consists of the following steps:

1. *Estimation of the time-frequency energy density for single trials.* The matching pursuit estimate was presented in the previous section. In the following section we will also discuss the performance of the spectrogram and scalogram.
2. *Delineation of the smallest time-frequency areas—called resels, from* resolution elements*—for which the statistical significance of energy changes will be assessed.* Resels are the resolution elements that determine the size of regions in which the hypothesis of no significant change of energy density (in relation to the reference epoch) will be tested. It determines the time-frequency resolution

of delineating the areas of significant energy changes. However, as can be expected, resels that are too small result in a noisy picture and less compact area of significance. Following the conclusions of [7], we use resels for which the product of the time and frequency dimensions gives $\frac{1}{2}$.

3. *Choice of the statistics for the null hypothesis of no change in a given resel,* as compared to the reference epoch in the same frequency. To validate the null hypothesis of no change in the average energy in a given resel with respect to the reference period, we can use any standard test for the difference of the means of two unequal groups. However, we must take into account possibly nonnormal distributions of the energy estimates. In the first approach [7], application of assumption-free resampling statistics (see [8]) resulted in computationally intensive procedures. A later study [9] proved that application of the Box-Cox transformation [10] to each resel's data gives a good approximation of the normal distribution, allowing for application of fast parametric statistics.

4. *Correction of the probability threshold for multiple comparisons.* Simultaneous testing in many resels implies facing the issue of multiple comparisons. To illustrate the problem, let's consider null hypothesis of no energy change in 20 *independent* time-frequency locations, tested at the significance level $\alpha = 5\%$. From the very definition of the significance level, we should expect approximately 1 in every 20 tests to indicate a statistically significant change even if the null hypothesis is correct. The simplest remedy to this problem is so-called Bonferroni correction. It divies the significance level of the individual tests by their number (i.e., each of the 20 tests should be performed with a significance level $\alpha/20 = 0.0025$).

   However, signals' energies estimated at neighboring time-frequency positions are not independent. Direct application of the Bonferroni correction in this case would result in very conservative tests,[2] which most probably would indicate no significant changes at all—with hundreds or thousands of resels tested simultaneously for changes, the significance level required for a single test would be extremely small. There are several ways to deal with the issue of multiple comparisons. Following [7], we apply the framework of False Discovery Rate (FDR, [11]). FDR gives the expected ratio of the number of resels with erroneously assigned significance to the total number of resels revealing significant changes. Setting FDR at 5% gives a possibility that 1 in 20 resels indicating changes may be actually insignificant.

2 In other words, the actual tests would be performed with a much lower α than assumed.

Mathematical and technical details of these steps are given in Chapter 15. Results of analysis of 57 artifact-free EEG trials from a standard fingertapping experiment [12] are presented in Plate 6. The first panel (a) of this figure presents a complete average map of energy density, calculated in the same way as the map from Plate 5.[3] Vertical lines mark the time epoch chosen as the reference and the instant of the event (in this case voluntary finger movement). The next panel (b) imposes quantization of energy density into resels. Panel (c) gives ERD/ERS calculated as the ratio of each resel's average energy to the average energy in the corresponding frequency, calculated for the whole reference epoch. Panel (d) presents the average values of ERD/ERS for only those resels, for which the earlier procedure indicated statistically significant changes; nonsignificant resels are marked in green.

Plate 6(e) presents the high-resolution map of ERD/ERS, calculated with the maximum resolution of the energy map. Finally, in panel (f) these high-resolution ERD and ERS are presented only within the area of resels revealing statistically significant changes of energy in relation to the reference epoch.

10.4 OTHER ESTIMATES OF SIGNAL'S ENERGY DENSITY

The MP-based procedure, presented in the previous section, was neither the first nor the only one proposed for the presentation of the complete time-frequency picture of event-related changes.

In 1993 Makeig proposed time-varying Fourier spectra, that he termed event-related spectral perturbation [13], for describing the auditory event-related dynamics of the EEG spectrum. Such an exploratory approach, free of a priori assumptions on fixed frequency bands, has been widely used in recent years. Apart from the time-varying spectra, equivalent to short-time Fourier transform (i.e., spectrogram described in Section 4.1), different methods are used for the estimation of the time-frequency density of signal energy, for example smoothed Wigner-Ville distributions [14, 15] and continuous wavelet transforms [16, 17]. These transforms, discussed briefly in Chapter 4, estimate the same quantity. However, the actual results, obtained for the same datasets via application of different estimates, vary depending on both the chosen method as well as the parameters chosen for a particular application.

3 For the sake of clarity, this distribution is presented in logarithmic scale, since otherwise the low-frequency, high-energy structures (we present the distribution starting from 0 Hz) would saturate the color scale. In further computations, the actual (linear) values of energy are used.

For example, as presented in Figure 4.2, different settings of the length of the analysis window in a spectrogram result in different properties of the estimate computed for the same signal. A spectrogram gives the best representation of these structures for which the time span is similar to the length of the analysis window. Correspondingly, choosing different wavelets for the scalogram also results in slightly different pictures, as exemplified in Figure 4.8.[4] Finally, the Wigner-Ville transform in signal analysis is practically never used in its raw form, as presented in Figure 4.9. Different kinds of smoothing kernels, reflecting different tradeoffs between the time and frequency resolutions, are applied in the hope of expressing optimally the structure of a given signal (see, for example, [18]).

These more or less arbitrary choices may produce a significant noise (or bias) in the results obtained using different methods and settings. In extreme cases it may even exceed the inherent, unavoidable noise present in the data, due, for example, to the great intersubject variability of EEG. This situation makes comparison of different studies difficult and reduces the value of neurophysiological conclusions drawn from these works. On the other hand, it is hard to judge a priori which of the estimators is "better" when analyzing signals of unknown content in the absence of well-defined criteria.

Plate 7 illustrates the performance of different estimates of time-frequency energy density, based upon an example analysis of ERD/ERS in ECoG data from a subject who underwent surgical implantation of subdural electrode grids over left frontoparietal cortical regions. The subject was asked to clench his right fist in response to a visual cue consisting of a picture of a fist on a video monitor. The subject clenched his fist while the visual cue was present (duration = 3 seconds) and relaxed his fist when the cue was replaced by a fixation point [19, 20]. The middle column of Plate 7 presents statistically significant ERD/ERS, corresponding to Plate 6 (f), calculated as described in Section 10.3.[5] Estimates of energy density in rows A, B, and C of Plate 7 were obtained, respectively, from the spectrogram (STFT), scalogram (continuous wavelet transform, CWT) and matching pursuit (MP) decomposition. The width of the spectrogram window, as well as the parameter governing the effective width of the analyzing wavelet, were

4 Figure 4.8 presents the simpler case of the discrete wavelet transform, while in the latter examples of the scalogram the continuous wavelet transform (CWT) will be used. These general conclusions hold for both the discrete and continuous versions.

5 The only difference is that statistics for single resels in Plate 6 were assessed by computationally intensive assumption-free resampling tests, while in Plate 7 a standard t-test was used after the Box-Cox transformation of data (Section 15.5). As proven in [9], as long as the normalization yields satisfactory approximation of normal distribution, differences in results are marginal.

chosen empirically to obtain clear pictures for this particular signal. On the contrary, MP estimates were obtained from a standard decomposition (13.7).

The MP algorithm does not rely on a priori settings related to the time-frequency resolution. As the only nonstandard setting, we may quote a larger than usual number of iterations, that is, the number M of functions included in signal expansion (13.11). It is needed to account for the weak structures in high frequencies. However, such a setting increases only the computational cost of the procedure and may be universally used in cases when relatively weak structures, like the high-frequency gamma oscillations, are of interest. Also, application of the coherence criterion (Section 13.7) should result in the automatic choice of an appropriate number of waveforms. These issues are discussed in Chapter 7.

The right and left columns of Plate 7 present a zoomed area of interest. We observe that in the maps derived from MP decomposition (row C), the significant regions are most compact, and the magnitude of ERD/ERS is the greatest. This is because the MP adapts representation to the structures present in the signal, does not require predetermined dependencies between time and frequency, and does not include cross-terms. These reasons may lead to more localized features in the time-frequency plane.

In the spectrogram (row A), there must be an a priori selection of constant time and frequency resolutions. Therefore, the structure of ERD/ERS consists of a composite of rectangular time-frequency pixels whose dimensions are determined by the selection of the method's fixed time-frequency resolution.

In the scalogram (row B), the frequency resolution is higher in low frequencies and lower in high frequencies. It results in a bias of the structure of ERD/ERS according to frequency. For example, high-gamma (>75 Hz) ERS occurs in structures that are elongated in the frequency dimension and abbreviated in the time dimension (row B, left column), whereas ERD/ERS in lower frequencies (<30 Hz, right column of row B) occur in structures that are elongated in the time dimension and compact in the frequency dimension. ERD/ERS structures at intermediate frequencies (30–50 Hz, right column of row B) have intermediate shapes with roughly equal time and frequency dimensions.

In contrast, the MP estimate produces ERD/ERS structures that do not appear to be consistently biased according to their occurrence in the frequency dimension. High-gamma ERS does occur over a broad range of frequencies, as shown with the spectrogram here and in a previous study [19], but the MP shows that this broadband response does not occur uniformly over all frequencies, as suggested by the spectrogram and the scalogram (Plate 7, C versus A and B, left column). Rather, the MP estimator indicates that high-gamma ERS consists of a collection of ERS responses at multiple frequencies, with variable latencies and energies. Likewise, the fine structures of alpha and beta ERD/ERS are quite different for MP versus the other estimators (Plate 7, C versus A and B, right column). In particular, the MP indicates that ERS in lower frequencies, associated with muscular relaxation, occurs in relatively broad bands and at relatively discrete times (row C, left column), compared with the structures indicated by the other estimators.

Based upon these considerations, we observe that final results of the determination of statistically significant ERD/ERS in the time-frequency plane depend on a number of parameters, including the following:

1. Choice of the estimator of time-frequency energy density and, except for the MP, empirical adjusting of its parameters;
2. Delineation of the reference epoch;
3. Size of time-frequency resels for statistics;
4. Statistical test used to assess the significance of changes in a single resel;
5. Choice of the framework for multiplicity correction.

However, as demonstrated in [7, 9], reasonable and statistically justified choices of parameters 2–5 result in procedures that delineate mostly similar time-frequency areas of the significant ERD/ERS. Some of these issues are discussed in more detail in Chapter 15.

Up to now, the choice of the energy density estimator and its parameters (1) remains the most arbitrary, yet crucial, step. It biases the time-frequency picture of ERD/ERS even if the parameters are empirically adopted to optimally represent a particular signal. In this light we may appreciate the built-in adaptivity of the MP algorithm, which results in freedom of the arbitrary choices that might significantly influence the results[6] and gives a representation with the time-frequency resolution automatically adopted to the local structures present in the signal.

Some of the discussed choices are illustrated in Figure 10.4, which presents one of the configuration windows from a software package implementing the discussed framework. The software package, which allows for experimenting with different settings of parameters, is freely available from http://eeg.pl. It implements all the calculations except for the MP decomposition, for which separate programs are available from http://eeg.pl/mp.

6 Except for a general knowledge of the proper application of MP (i.e., including enough waveforms in the decomposition and using large enough dictionary, as discussed in Chapter 7).

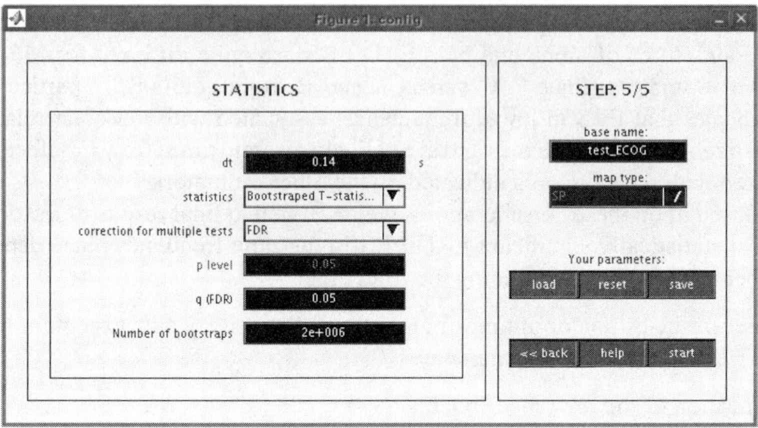

Figure 10.4 Some choices involved in the creation of the time-frequency maps of statistically significant ERD/ERS (as in Plates 6 and 7). This configuration window sets the time width of a resel used for calculating the statistical significance (frequency width will be adjusted so that $\Delta t \Delta f = \frac{1}{2}$), type of the statistics used for single-resel tests (bootstrapped t-statistics, permutation test, parametric t-test, parametric Z-test), correction for multiple comparisons (FDR, Bonferroni-Holmes, or none), significance or, if FDR was chosen, parameter q (Section 15.6), and the number of bootstrap repetitions for resampling procedures. The right panel indicates the chosen time-frequency estimate (MP, CWT, or spectrogram). The Matlab code of the software from which the screenshot was taken is freely available from http://eeg.pl.

References

[1] M. A. B. Brazier, *A History of the Electrical Activity of the Brain: The First Half-Century*, London: Pitman Medical Publishing, 1961.

[2] H. Berger, "Über das Elektrenkephalogramm des Menschen II," *J. Psychol. Neurol.*, vol. 40, 1930, pp. 160–179.

[3] A. Beck, "Die Ströme der Nervencentren," *Centerblatt für Physiologie*, vol. 4, 1890, pp. 572–573.

[4] G. Pfurtscheller and A. Arnibar, "Evaluation of Event-Related Desynchronization (ERD) Preceding and Following Voluntary Self-Paced Movements," *Electroencephalography and Clinical Neurophysiology*, vol. 46, 1979, pp. 128–146.

[5] P. J. Durka, et al., "Time-Frequency Microstructure of Event-Related Desynchronization and Synchronization," *Medical & Biological Engineering & Computing*, vol. 39, no. 3, 2001, pp. 315–321.

[6] G. Pfurtscheller and F. H. Lopes da Silva, "Event-Related EEG/MEG Synchronization and Desynchronization: Basic Principles," *Clinical Neurophysiology*, vol. 110, 1999, pp. 1842–1857.

[7] P. J. Durka, et al., "On the Statistical Significance of Event-Related EEG Desynchronization and Synchronization in the Time-Frequency Plane," *IEEE Transactions on Biomedical Engineering*, vol. 51, 2004, pp. 1167–1175.

[8] B. Efron and R. J. Tibshirani, *An Introduction to the Bootstrap*, London: Chapman & Hall, 1993.

[9] J. Żygierewicz, et al., "Computationally Efficient Approaches to Calculating Significant ERD/ERS Changes in the Time-Frequency Plane," *Journal of Neuroscience Methods*, vol. 145, no. 1–2, 2005, pp. 267–276.

[10] G. E. P. Box and D. R. Cox, "An Analysis of Transformations," *Journal of the Royal Statistical Society*, vol. 2, 1964, pp. 211–252.

[11] Y. Benjamini and Y. Yekutieli, "The Control of the False Discovery Rate Under Dependency," *Ann. Stat.*, vol. 29, 2001, pp. 1165–1188.

[12] J. Ginter Jr., et al., "Phase and Amplitude Analysis in Time-Frequency Space—Application to Voluntary Finger Movement," *Journal of Neuroscience Methods*, vol. 110, 2001, pp. 113–124.

[13] S. Makeig, "Auditory Event-Related Dynamics of the EEG Spectrum and Effects of Exposure to Tones," *Electroencephalography and Clinical Neurophysiology*, vol. 86, 1993, pp. 283–293.

[14] E. Rodriguez, et al., "Perception's Shadow: Long-Distance Synchronization of Human Brain Activity," *Nature*, vol. 397, 1999, pp. 430–433.

[15] J.-P. Lachaux, et al., "A Quantitative Study of Gamma-Band Activity in Human Intracranial Recordings Triggered by Visual Stimuli," *European Journal of Neuroscience*, vol. 12, 2000, pp. 2608–2622.

[16] O. Bertrand and C. Tallon-Baudry, "Oscillatory Gamma Activity in Humans: A Possible Role for Object Representation," *International Journal of Psychophysiology*, vol. 38, 2000, pp. 211–223.

[17] C. Tallon-Baudry, A. Kreiter, and O. Bertrand, "Sustained and Transient Oscillatory Responses in the Gamma and Beta Bands in a Visual Short-Term Memory Task in Humans," *Visual Neuroscience*, vol. 16, 1999, pp. 449–459.

[18] W. J. Williams, "Recent Advances in Time-Frequency Representations: Some Theoretical Foundations," in *Time Frequency and Wavelets in Biomedical Signal Processing*, M. Akay, (ed.), IEEE Press Series in Biomedical Engineering, New York: IEEE Press, 1997, pp. 3–44.

[19] N. E. Crone, et al., "Functional Mapping of Human Sensorimotor Cortex with Electrocorticigraphic Spectral Analysis II. Event-Related Synchronization in the Gamma Band," *Brain*, vol. 121, 1998, pp. 2301–2315.

[20] N. E. Crone, et al., "Functional Mapping of Human Sensorimotor Cortex with Electrocorticigraphic Spectral Analysis I. Alpha and Beta Event-Related Desynchronization," *Brain*, vol. 121, 1998, pp. 2271–2299.

Chapter 11

Selective Estimates of Energy

This chapter presents improvements in sensitivity that can be achieved in standard research and clinical paradigms by replacing previously applied spectral integrals with selective and sensitive MP-derived estimates of energy. Selectivity is based upon the general knowledge of investigated phenomena, which can be employed, for example, by incorporating the detailed definitions of relevant structures (as in Chapter 8).

In the previous chapter, we used matching pursuit decompositions solely for computation of the time-frequency estimates (maps) of signal energy density—they were used in exactly the same way as the maps obtained from a spectrogram or scalogram. MP-based estimates displayed some advantages, like high resolution and adaptivity of the time-frequency resolution to the local properties of the signal. However, parametric description of the signal structures underlying the construction of these maps was not explored in this approach. This chapter presents how we can profit from this unique feature of the MP in paradigms, which are traditionally based upon estimation of energy in fixed time-frequency regions (e.g., frequency bands); selectivity of MP-derived estimates of energy of relevant structures was also briefly suggested in Figure 8.8.

Let us recall the uncertainty principle in signal analysis (Section 3.2). It states that every function (i.e., every signal and every structure present in a signal) has nonzero widths in both time and frequency domains. The product of these widths is bound to exceed a certain constant, which causes the omnipresent tradeoff in the time-frequency resolution: the better the time localization (i.e., smaller time width) of a waveform, the wider its spread in frequency. For now let us concentrate on the fact that these spreads are nonzero. Theoretically, we may say that an infinite sine wave has no uncertainty (zero width) in frequency and infinite width (uncertainty) in time. Similarly Dirac's delta has perfect localization in time and infinite spread in frequency domain. But in practice we deal with finite epochs and finite resolutions. So, for example, when talking about a Gabor function with frequency of 15 Hz, we should correctly speak about the frequency *center* of a function, since its energy will also be spread below and above 15 Hz (see Figure 6.1).

What happens when we compute the spectral energy of a signal in given frequency band? Most of the energy contained in this band, say between 12 and 14 Hz, will be indeed contributed by the structures with frequency centers lying within that range. However, tails of energy distributions of the structures with frequency centers slightly above 14 Hz and slightly below 12 Hz will also contribute to this integral. On the other hand, tails of energy distributions of the structures originating between 12 and 14 Hz will fall outside this interval and hence will not contribute to the spectral integral. To estimate exactly and selectively only the energy carried by the structures with frequency centers between 12 and 14 Hz, we need their explicit parameterization, like the MP expansion. This situation is illustrated in Figure 11.1.

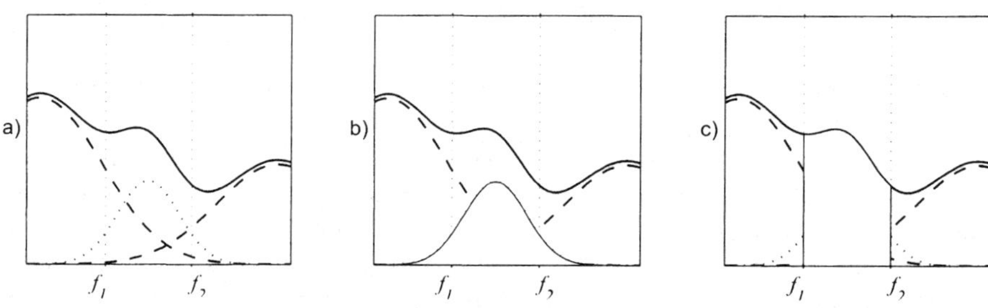

Figure 11.1 The difference between the spectral integral from f_1 to f_2 (shaded in (c)) and the actual power carried by structure(s) with frequency center(s) lying within this interval (b). Black solid line—spectrum resulting from the presence of all three structures. Their spectra are plotted separately with dotted and dashed lines in (a). (b) Power carried by the structure with a frequency center between f_1 and f_2 (gray). (c) Spectral integral from f_1 to f_2 (gray). We observe that part of the energy originating within the interval spreads outside it, while part of the energy of structures originating at outside frequencies contributes to the power integrated within the interval. Explicit parameterization of signal structures, like the MP expansion, allows for computation of estimates corresponding to the gray area in (b).

11.1 ERD/ERS ENHANCEMENT

Let us return to the time-frequency estimates of event-related gamma synchronization (ERS), presented in Section 10.2. Classical estimation of ERD/ERS, presented in Figure 10.2, relied on estimating the energy content in predefined frequency bands, which were chosen via a trial-and-error procedure. Application of the high-resolution MP estimates of energy density resulted in a significant increase of the gamma ERS, calculated for the same frequency bands (Figure 10.3). This increase indicates an improvement of sensitivity in respect to this parameter.

However, increased sensitivity was not the only gain from the application of a time-frequency estimate: it also allowed for a presentation of a complete picture of the average energy density, as in Plate 5. Let us recall the upper part of this picture, containing gamma activity. We observe that the increase of the energy before the movement onset occurs mostly between 35 and 38 Hz. Therefore, we may obtain a more sensitive measure of this premovement gamma synchronization by selecting this band, instead of the previously chosen 36–40 Hz.

Optimization of the frequency band still does not exhaust the list of possible improvements. We may also employ the observation from Figure 11.1, and, instead of calculating the whole energy in the band, we may selectively take into account only the energy of the structures with frequency centers lying in the chosen interval. Gain introduced by these improvements results in doubled sensitivity to the gamma ERS, as illustrated in Figure 11.2.

11.2 PHARMACO EEG

Fourier transform is one of the very few—if not the only—signal processing method widely adopted in the practice of EEG analysis. Its acceptance is due to a long record of applications (it was first applied to EEG analysis in 1932 [1]), fast numerical implementations (since the introduction of the fast Fourier transform in 1965 [2]), and relatively simple interpretation of results.

One of the paradigms established for quantifying drug effects on the central nervous system, called pharmaco EEG, relies on Fourier estimates—see http://www.internationalpharmacoeeggroup.org, the home page of the International Pharmaco-EEG Society. Spectral powers are calculated in frequency bands corresponding to standard EEG rhythms, and their changes under the influence of drugs—called drug profiles—are related to the actions of particular groups of drugs.

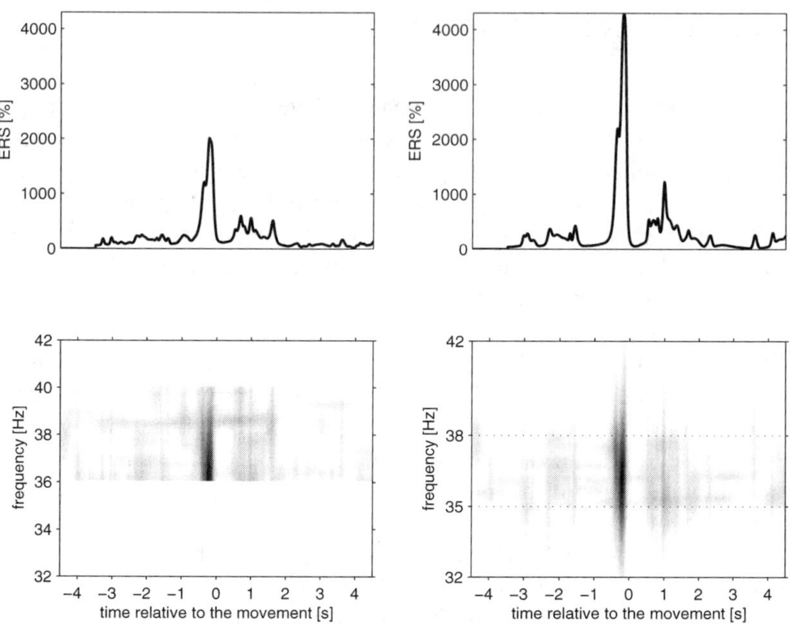

Figure 11.2 Estimation of the gamma ERS from the MP estimates. Left column: as in Figure 10.3, energy in the band 36–40 Hz is integrated to produce the ERS curve in the upper row, which presents the increase of the energy relative to the reference epoch, chosen between -4.5 and -3.5 seconds. Right column: time-frequency energy density of structures with frequency centers lying between 35 and 38 Hz (lower panel), and the corresponding ERS curve (above). Computed from the same dataset as Figures 10.2 and 10.3, and Plate 5.

For sleep-inducing drugs, changes of power in delta (δ), theta (θ), and sigma (σ) bands during overnight sleep are usually considered. Spectral integrals in the delta and sigma bands estimate the power of slow waves and sleep spindles (definitions of these structures were given in Section 8.2). However, as presented at the beginning of this chapter in Figure 11.1, these estimates incorporate a lot of noise. It results from including the energy of structures lying outside the relevant intervals, and at the same time neglecting tails of energy distributions of the relevant structures. The possibility of a selective estimation of the energy of structures, originating within a chosen frequency band, was investigated in the previous section. In this section we will combine this approach with another major advantage of adaptive approximations, explored in Chapter 8. We recall that MP decomposition allows us to select relevant structures based not only upon their frequencies, but also amplitudes, time widths, and so forth. We can use this information for picking the relevant waveforms from the MP expansion of signals, and then, for the selected structures, compute a selective estimator corresponding to the spectral power. Due to an exact estimation of the energy of relevant structures only, we expect an improvement in sensitivity as compared to the spectral integrals.

In the following, we verify these expectations on a standard dataset, collected according to the paradigm used in pharmaco EEG studies of drug influence on sleep. It contains 21 all-night recordings of 7 paid volunteers: 3 males and 4 females (mean age: 33.6, SD$\pm$5.4, range 25–41 years) with no psychiatric, medical, or sleep disorders. All participants were required to be free of any prescription or nonprescription drugs for at least 2 weeks before the study. Sleep was recorded during 3 blocks of 3 consecutive nights, with at least 2 weeks interval [3].

For each of these subjects, polysomnograms were recorded after administering at bedtime zolpidem (10 mg), midazolam (7.5 mg), and placebo in random order according to a double-blind, crossover design. Polygraphic monitoring consisted of EEG activity collected from 21 electrodes, according to the international 10–20 system, electrooculogram (EOG) from two channels, and submentalis electromyogram. Filters were set between 0.15 and 30.0 Hz. The impedance at each electrode was below 5,000 ohms. Sleep stages and artifacts were identified visually (stages according to the standardized manual [4]). For the analysis presented in this chapter, we used artifact-free epochs from derivation C3–A2.

For the standard pharmaco EEG, it is enough to define the spectral bands of interest; in [3] the following definitions were assumed: δ 0.75–4 Hz, θ 4–8 Hz, and σ 12–14 Hz (lower frequency for δ activity was raised to avoid the low-frequency artifacts). Since we are using the MP parameterization, we can also employ some extra information on the relevant structures, like the minimum amplitude or time width. This kind of information is often available in the classical definitions of structures (e.g., sleep spindles or slow waves), formulated for the sake of standardization of visual EEG analysis (see [4]). Correspondence between the visual detection of waveforms present in sleep EEG and their MP parameterization was explored in Chapter 8. Criteria used in this study [3] are summarized in Table 11.1. In addition to these criteria, for the analysis of slow wave activity (δ) only data from stages 3 and 4 was used; for the θ band data from all sleep stages was used, and for sleep spindles (σ) only data from sleep stage 2 was used.

Table 11.1
Frequency Bands and Parameters Defining Relevant Structures Used in [3] and Figures 11.3–11.6.

	Frequency	Time Duration	Min. Amplitude
δ (slow waves)	0.75–4 Hz	0.5–∞ s.	75 μV
θ	4–8 Hz	—	30 μV
σ (sleep spindles)	12–14 Hz	0.5–2.5 s.	15 μV

To validate the agreement with the previously established paradigm, spectral estimates of energy in the relevant bands were calculated first.[1] Figure 11.3 presents FFT spectra in the sigma band, calculated for the C3–A2 derivation of each of the analyzed recordings. Plots are organized in columns, corresponding—from the left—to the nights after administering placebo, zolpidem, and midazolam. Each row contains analysis of recordings of one of the subjects, from now on referred to as #1–#7: from subject #1 in the upper row, through #2 in the second from the top, and so on up to #7 in the bottom row. On the right of each plot, total spectral power in the sigma band is given in μV^2. Below this value we quote its mean squared error (MSE) and the total time of qualifying epochs used in calculations. We recall that the spectral estimate of power in given band was calculated separately for each 4-second epoch and averaged, which allows the computation of an estimate of its variance. In the middle and right columns, corresponding to the nights after zolpidem and midazolam, relative change of power—related to the night after placebo—is given in percent above these numbers.

We observe a general increase of power in the σ band in the signals recorded after either of the administered drugs, in relation to the night after the placebo of the same subject. It is in line with previous works reporting such behavior for different benzodiazepine receptor agonists [5–7]. However, recording of subject #7 (lower row) for the night after midazolam (right column) indicates a weak reverse trend, that is, a very little (4%) decrease of the power estimated from spectral integrals. This may be due to the very low activity in the σ band of this patient. In a case when the phenomenon in question is weak, fluctuations may mask the investigated effect

1 For calculation of the spectral estimates of energy, artifact-free data from relevant stages was further divided into 4-second epochs. For each of these epochs, spectral density of energy was estimated as a squared magnitude of discrete Fourier transform of the epoch multiplied by 4-second Hamming window. From this estimate, a spectral integral in the relevant range (Table 11.1) was extracted separately for each epoch.

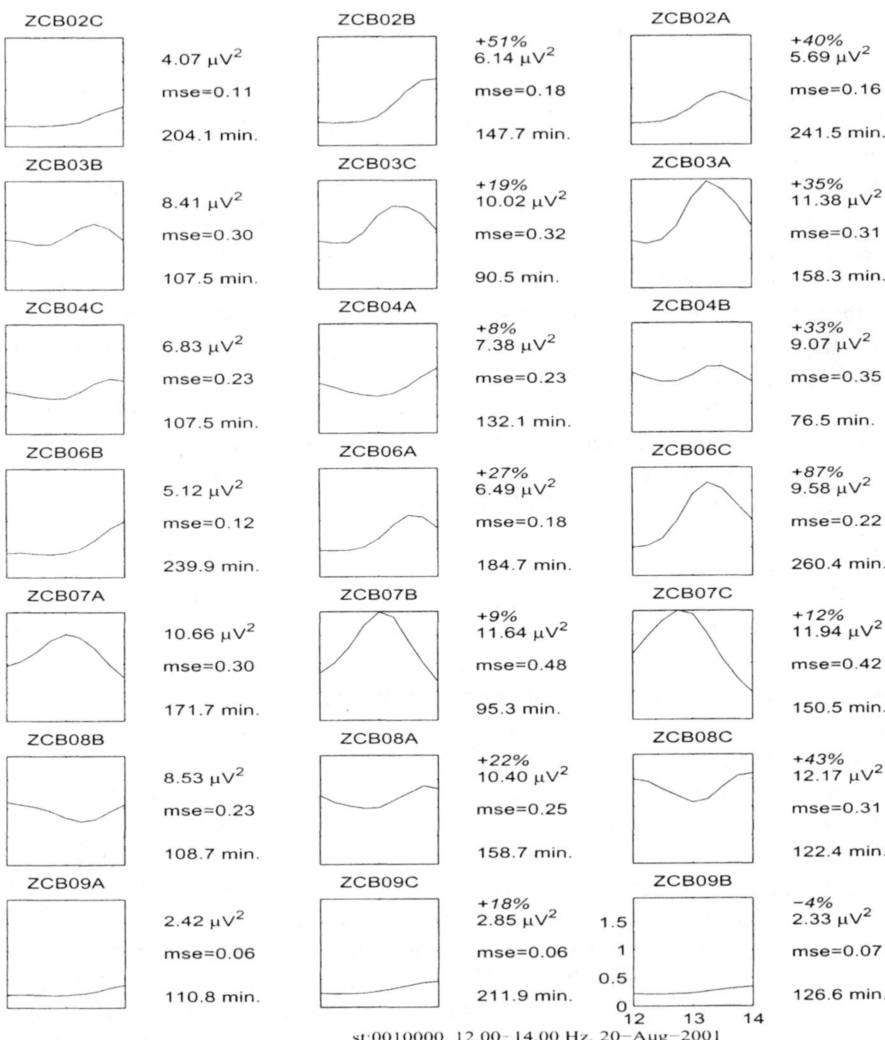

Figure 11.3 Spectra in the σ band. Columns (from the left) correspond to nights after placebo, zolpidem, and midazolam. Each row represents one subject (code above each box), in the text referred to as #1–#7 (from top). Values on the right of each plot are described in the caption of Figure 11.5.

to such an extent. Within the proposed framework, we may get rid of the part of these fluctuations that results from low selectivity of the spectral estimate.

Figure 11.4 presents estimates of power carried only by the structures conforming to all the criteria from Table 11.1 for sleep spindles (i.e., also conditions on the time length and minimum amplitude). Plots for each patient and drug are organized in rows and columns in exactly the same order as in Figure 11.3. Instead of spectral powers between 12 and 14 Hz, these plots present each of the structures classified as a sleep spindle as a dot in the frequency-amplitude coordinates. Total power of sleep spindles, given on the right in μV^2, is now estimated from the sum of the energies of all these structures. Energies were normalized per time unit. Also, note that the energy is not exactly equivalent to amplitude. A structure of the same amplitude but longer in time will carry more energy.

Apart from the total power, on the right of each plot we also quote some parameters inaccessible from the spectral estimates—from the top: average number of structures per minute, their mean amplitude and its variance, and the mean frequency with variance. In calculating this mean, frequencies were weighted by the amplitudes.

Information from Figures 11.3 and 11.4 is summarized in Table 11.2. It compares changes of power of sleep spindles in recordings after administration of zolpidem and midazolam, as related to nights after placebo, estimated in two different ways. Rows labelled "FT" contain the percent of changes calculated as the ratio of spectral estimates of energy in the sigma band (from Figure 11.3), while rows labelled "MP" give this ratio for the MP-based estimates of power of sleep spindles (presented in Figure 11.4). We observe that MP-based selective estimates reveal on the average about twice higher sensitivity to the drug-induced changes of energy. Also, the only case in which the FFT estimates were obscured by fluctuations so much that they presented a reverse trend (marked bold in Table 11.2) within the MP-based framework is resolved in concordance with all the other cases as well as the expectations from previous studies.

Figures 11.5 and 11.6 present the same reports, discussed earlier for sleep spindles, but computed for delta waves. A summary of the relative changes of power in δ band is given in Table 11.3. Figure 11.5 contains plots of the δ band power, organized and labeled in exactly the same way as in Figure 11.3; the only difference is that the spectral integral was this time calculated in the 0.75–4-Hz range. A consistent general trend presents a decrease of power in the sigma band, which is again in line with the previously published research [5–7]. However, two subjects (#6 and #7, two lower rows) exhibit overall low activity in the δ band. Fourier analysis of one of these recordings—subject #6 after midazolam, middle

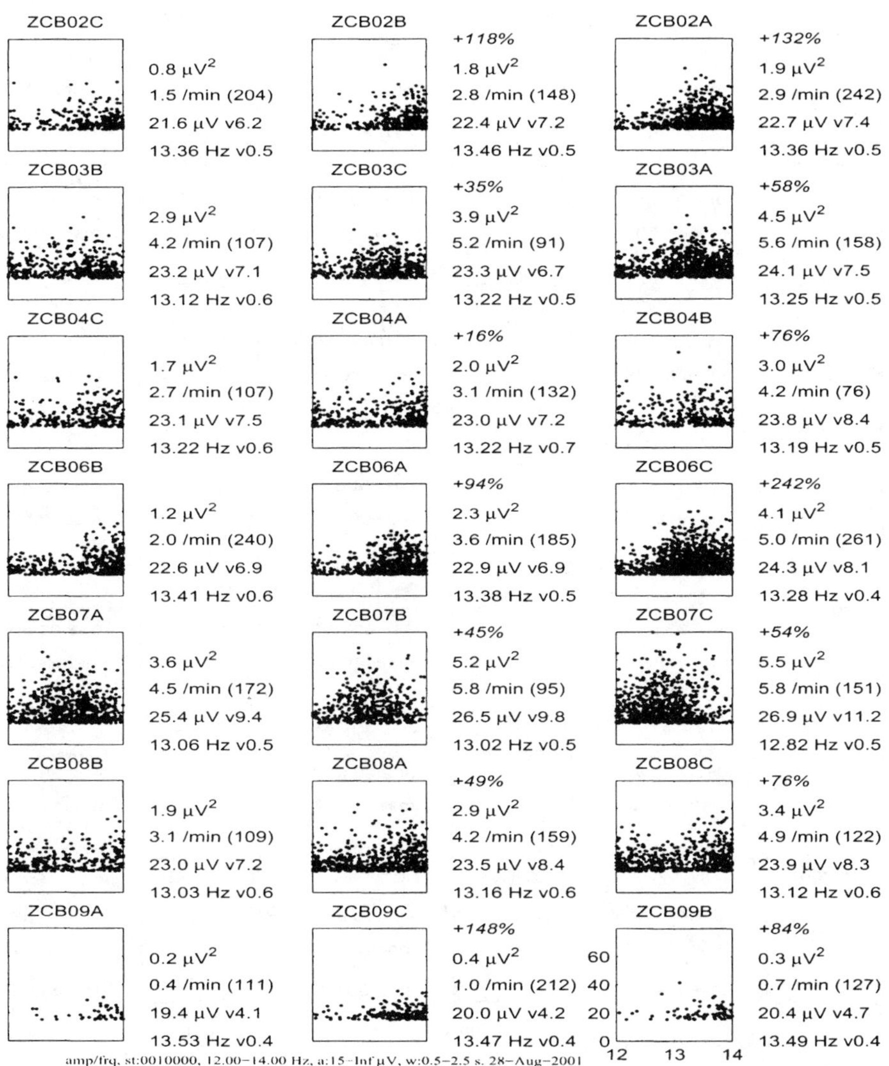

Figure 11.4 Each box corresponds to one overnight recording, as in Figure 11.3. Within boxes, black dots represent structures classified as sleep spindles—according to criteria from Table 11.1—in the frequency (horizontal, Hz) versus amplitude (vertical, μV) coordinates.

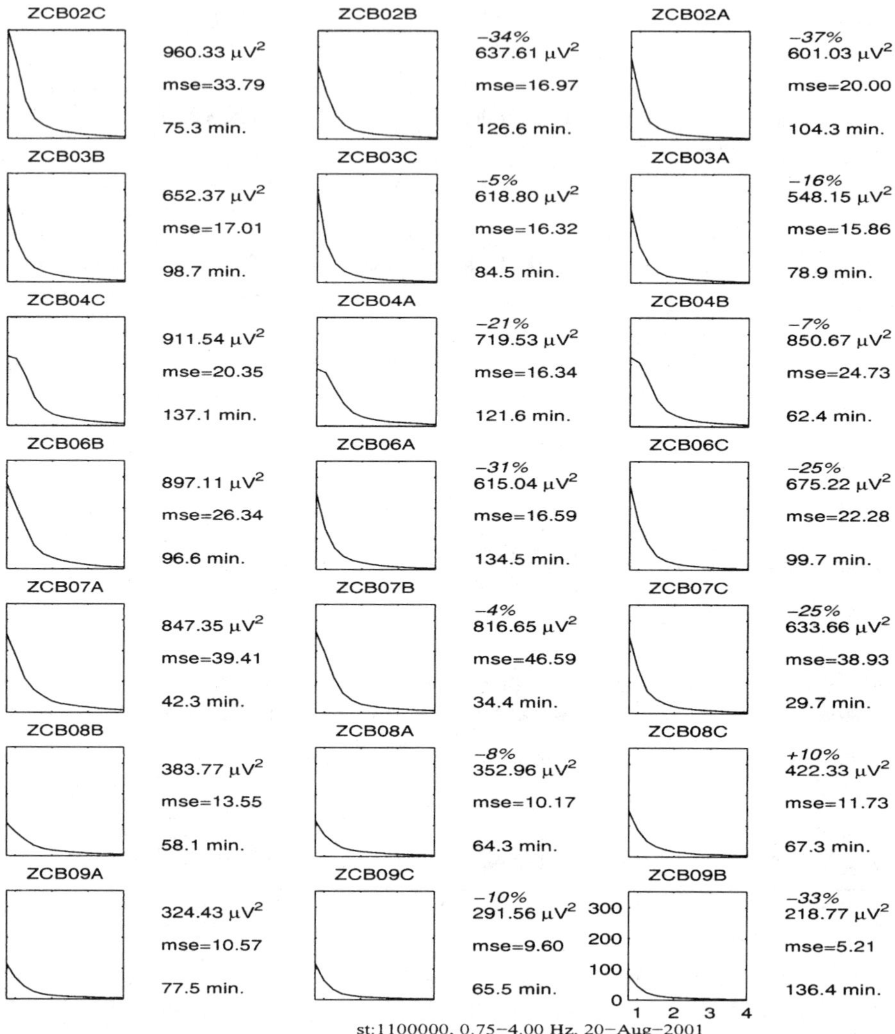

Figure 11.5 Spectra for the δ band, organized as in Figure 11.3. On the right of each plot, power (μV^2), its mean square error (mse), and total time of epochs from which the estimate was calculated, are given. For the nights after zolpidem and midazolam (middle and right columns), the percent change of power (related to the night after placebo) is given above the quoted numbers.

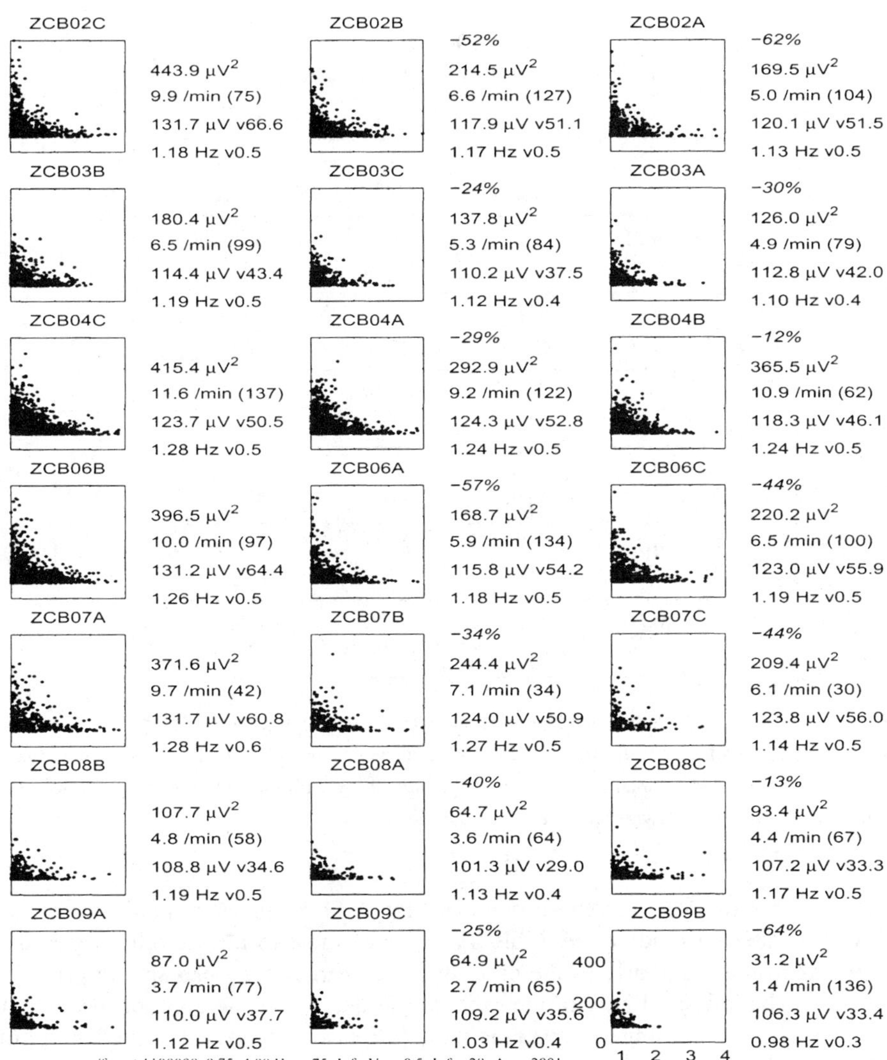

Figure 11.6 Slow waves selected from the MP parameterization according to criteria from Table 11.1. Plots and descriptions are organized as in Figure 11.4.

Table 11.2
Changes of Power in the Sigma Band

Subject	Estimate	Zolpidem	Midazolam
#1	FT	+51%	+40%
	MP	+115%	+134%
#2	FT	+19%	+35%
	MP	+37%	+56%
#3	FT	+8%	+33%
	MP	+20%	+76%
#4	FT	+27%	+87%
	MP	+95%	+242%
#5	FT	+9%	+12%
	MP	+41%	+51%
#6	FT	+22%	+43%
	MP	+47%	+80%
#7	FT	+18%	**–4%**
	MP	+154%	+68%

Percentages for the nights after zolpidem and midazolam were calculated as ratios of energies, relative to the nights after placebo, estimated as: (1) spectral integrals from 12 to 14 Hz (upper value in each cell, labeled "FT") and (2) total energy of sleep spindles, chosen from MP decompositions based upon criteria from Table 11.1 (lower row of each cell, labeled "MP").

column, second row from the bottom in Figure 11.5—gives a small increase of power (printed in boldface in Table 11.3), in contrast to all the other cases and previous results. Similarly to the case discussed earlier for sleep spindles, it may be due to the low sensitivity of the spectral estimate in the situation of low signal-to-noise ratio. According to expectation, the MP-based analysis presented in Figure 11.6 resolves this case in line with the other results.

As for the theta band, MP-based estimates did not differ significantly from the FFT, so results for θ are not presented here (these results are summarized in [3]). Lack of an improvement in θ is most probably due to the fact that the filters defined in Table 11.1 do not contain much specific information for these structures, in particular there were no restrictions on time width. This result indicates that the

Table 11.3

Changes of Power in the Delta Band

Subject	Estimate	Zolpidem	Midazolam
#1	FT	–34%	–37%
	MP	–51%	-63%
#2	FT	–5%	–16%
	MP	–24%	–30%
#3	FT	–21%	–7%
	MP	–30%	–16%
#4	FT	–31%	–25%
	MP	–57%	–44%
#5	FT	–4%	–25%
	MP	–21%	–44%
#6	FT	–8%	**+10%**
	MP	–39%	–14%
#7	FT	–10%	–33%
	MP	–27%	–62%

Percentages for the nights after zolpidem and midazolam were calculated as ratios of energies, relative to the nights after placebo, estimated as: (1) spectral integrals from 0.75 to 4 Hz (upper value in each cell, labeled "FT") and (2) total energy of slow waves, chosen from MP decompositions based upon criteria from Table 11.1 (lower row of each cell, labeled "MP").

extra information about the relevant structures contained in Table 11.1 plays a more important role than sole restriction of the estimates to the structures originating within the selected frequency band (effect illustrated in Figure 11.1).

Finally, observed differences were tested statistically. Table 11.4 gives results of two tests. Statistics were applied to the average energies for each subject under a given condition (placebo, zolpidem, and midazolam), treated as three matched vectors with seven values (seven subjects) each. The overall hypothesis of no difference between columns (i.e., between the nights after administering either of the drugs) was assessed by Friedmann's nonparametric two-way analysis of variance [8]. To find out which particular pairs exhibited possible differences,

Wilcoxon signed rank test [8] was computed for differences between all three pairs separately.

Table 11.4

Values of p for the Null Hypothesis of No Change in the Nights After Different Drugs

δ (slow waves, 0.75–4 Hz)			
	F	pl–zo	pl–mi
FT	0.021	+	0.031
pow.	0.005	+	+
n/min	0.005	+	+
freq.	0.006	0.031	+

σ (sleep spindles, 12–14 Hz)			
	F	pl–zo	pl–mi
FT	0.018	+	0.031
pow.	0.021	+	+
n/min	0.002	+	+
freq.	0.46	0.69	0.56

Columns "F": Friedmann's nonparametric two-way analysis of variance, testing differences between the nights after placebo, zolpidem, and midazolam. Columns "pl–zo" and "pl–mi": Wilcoxon signed rank test for nights after placebo and zolplidem and placebo and midazolam, correspondingly. No significant differences were found between the nights after zolpidem and midazolam. Statistics computed for spectral estimates of energy (row "FT") and parameters derived from MP decompositions: mean power ("pow."), number of occurrences per minute ("n/min"), and mean frequency ("freq."). Results presented for the δ (left) and σ (right table) bands. Plus (+) marks the value of $p = 0.0156$, minimum in Wilcoxon test for paired vectors of size 7.

The first two rows of Table 11.4 confirm what's easily seen in Tables 11.2 and 11.3. The power of structures selected in the respective bands reveals changes consistent with spectral integrals, usually with better significance. However, as presented in Figures 11.4 and 11.6, MP parameterization allows us to compute, from the same decompositions, a multitude of different parameters. In this study we tested the average frequency, weighted by amplitudes, and number of occurrences per minute of sleep spindles and slow waves (two lower rows of Table 11.4). Of these two, the number of occurrences per minute revealed statistical significances (third row of Table 11.4) fully consistent with those of the changes in mean energy, for both sleep spindles and slow waves. This indicates that the changes in power, carried by the slow waves and sleep spindles, seem to be caused by the change in the number of their occurrences rather than average increase or decrease of their amplitudes, since changes in the average amplitudes were not significant. However, to evaluate this hypothesis rigorously, we would have to also take into account the average length and/or power carried by these structures, since a structure of the same amplitude with a longer time span carries more energy. Such issues would be extremely difficult to address within the classical paradigm, relying, for example, on spectral powers; hereby they appear as just another report from the database of parameters of automatically detected structures.

Finally, the last row on the left in Table 11.4 reveals statistical significance of a completely new effect, which was not reported in the previous works: a significant, drug-induced change of the mean frequency of slow waves. From the numbers given in Figure 11.6 we read that this change is a small, yet statistically significant, decrease. Again, this observation gives an example of an effect completely elusive to the previously applied methods.

References

[1] G. Dietsch, "Fourier Analyse von Elektroenzephalogrammen des Menschen," *Pflügers Arch. Ges. Physiol.*, vol. 230, 1932, pp. 106–112.

[2] J. W. Cooley and J. W. Tukey, "An Algorithm for the Machine Calculation of Complex Fourier Series," *Mathematics of Computation*, vol. 19, 1965, pp. 297–301.

[3] P. J. Durka, et al., "Adaptive Time-Frequency Parametrization in Pharmaco EEG," *Journal of Neuroscience Methods*, vol. 117, 2002, pp. 65–71.

[4] A. Rechtschaffen and A. Kales, (eds.), *A Manual of Standardized Terminology, Techniques and Scoring System for Sleep Stages in Human Subjects*, Number 204 in National Institutes of Health Publications, U.S. Government Printing Office, Washington, D.C., 1968.

[5] D. P. Brunner, et al., "Effect of Zolpidem on Sleep and Sleep EEG Spectra in Healthy Young Men," *Psychopharmacology*, vol. 104, 1991, pp. 1–5.

[6] B. Feige, et al., "Independent Sleep EEG Slow-wave and Spindle Band Dynamics Associated with 4 Weeks of Continuous Application of Short Half-Life Hypnotics in Healthy Subjects," *Clinical Neurophysiology*, vol. 110, 1999, pp. 1965–1974.

[7] L. Trachsel, et al., "Effect of Zopiclone and Midazolam on Sleep and EEG Spectra in a Phase-Advanced Sleep Schedule," *Neuropsychopharmacology*, vol. 3, 1990, pp. 11–18.

[8] *Statistic Toolbox User's Guide (Version 3)*, The MathWorks, Inc., November 2000.

Chapter 12

Spatial Localization of Cerebral Sources

This chapter presents improvement in localization of cerebral sources of EEG activity, brought by selective parameterization of relevant structures by the multichannel version of matching pursuit combined with EEG inverse solutions.

As mentioned in the Introduction, for more than 70 years EEG has been the most direct trace of thought that we can measure. Recently it seems to be losing importance in favor of new brain imaging techniques, which offer results in terms of easily interpretable images. Obviously, no clinician or neurophysiologist would analyze raw signals from the fMRI or PET sensors.

However, there exist a wide class of techniques, called EEG inverse solutions, that provide 3-D images of cerebral current densities, estimated from multichannel EEG. We will briefly recall some of their basic properties and limitations. As a partial solution to their inherent sensitivity to noise present in EEG traces, before the application of an EEG inverse solution we perform multichannel matching pursuit decomposition (presented in detail in Section 13.12). This scheme allows us to use the same frameworks for selection of the relevant structures, as discussed and verified in the monochannel case (see Chapters 8 and 9), and improves stability of the localization.

12.1 EEG INVERSE SOLUTIONS

Several attempts were directed at relating the structures, known from the EEG traces, to the anatomical locations of their cerebral generators. Unfortunately, this so-called EEG inverse problem is ill-posed (in the sense of Hadamard [1]). In relation to the localization of cerebral sources of electric activity, measured from the skull, it means that:

1. The solution is nonunique, because there is an infinity of possible electric current density distributions in the brain that may generate the same potential on the scalp surface. This ambiguity of the underlying static electromagnetic problem was proved by Helmholtz in 1853 [2].
2. Small changes in the input data (that is, EEG measured at the electrodes) may lead to big changes in the solution (spatial localization of sources).

Choosing a unique solution requires prior information, independent of the EEG data, which is usually arbitrary choices of additional constraints. There can be different kinds of constraints, the most used of which are of anatomical and physical-mathematical nature. The former consists basically of restricting the solution to some physiologically supported area, which can be a particular structure or the whole gray matter. The latter varies from considering the solution to be a sum of current dipoles to choosing the distributed solution with minimum norm or maximum smoothness. Solving an ill-posed problem by adding additional information about the solution was first treated by the Tikhonov regularization [3–5]. The Bayesian approach allows us to introduce a priori information in a natural and flexible way [6, 7].

According to constraints and algorithms used, different solutions are being promoted by different groups (e.g., LAURA, EPIFOCUS [8], ELECTRA [9] and LORETA [3], with variants such as sLORETA [10], VARETA [11], and Bayesian Model Averaging [7]). Just from the abundance of different solutions, one can see that the issue is complicated and provides far from stable conclusions, since none of the mentioned methods gives fully satisfactory results in all kinds of EEG data. In this regard, an inverse solution is preferred according to the case of study. Some of them are suitable for applications in which a small region of the brain is active (as is the case, for example, in evoked potential studies), and others when the current density is spread out in wider areas (e.g., spontaneous EEG, tumors, epilepsy). On the other hand, most of them, particularly LORETA, present usually physiologically noninterpretable sources, called ghost sources, and an inherent incapacity for recovering deep sources [7].

12.2 IS IT A TOMOGRAPHY?

Three-dimensional reconstruction of the current densities inside the brain, obtained from one of the previously mentioned inverse solutions, is commonly termed "brain electrical tomography" (BET). The term "tomography" is also explicitly present in the names of some of the most known EEG inverse solution methods (e.g., LORETA stands for "LOw Resolution Electromagnetic TomogrAphy"). However, if we adhere to this naming, we must accept that different tomographs[1] can provide significantly different images for the same case.

The common meaning of the word "tomography" is "a method of producing a three-dimensional image of the internal structures of a solid object (as the human body or the earth) by the observation and recording of the differences in the effects on the passage of waves of energy impinging on those structures."[2] In the techniques introduced after CT, information from a single plane (section) is obtained by varying gradients of magnetic fields (MRI) or moving the ring of detectors (PET). Although these techniques may not fall into the exact scope of the classical definition, related to X-rays, they employ the same scheme of reconstructing the image. Underlying physical processes provide robust information about sections, and 3-D images are created from these slices via separate mathematical procedure.

Physics governing the propagation of the electrical field does not allow for a selective measuring of slices, since changes of conductivity or potential outside the predetermined plane also influence the readings of electrodes lying in this plane. So, actually, the procedures applied in tomography and EEG inverse solutions are somehow reversed: in tomography we reconstruct a 3-D image by combining separately obtained slices, while inverse solutions compute the whole 3-D distribution, which can be later presented as slices.

Different mechanisms employed in forming images imply the major difference between tomography and EEG inverse solutions. In true tomographies, known accuracy of physical processes involved in separate measurements of planes or beams, and stability of the mathematics employed in tomographic reconstructions, prevent the possibility of two different machines (or algorithms) giving significantly different locations of the same structure. In this sense, EEG inverse solutions are not as reliable as medical imaging techniques, and their applications must be preceded by a correct understanding of the physical and mathematical basis needed

1 Or even the same "tomographs"—in this case, algorithms for EEG inverse solution—with different settings of parameters.

2 Meriam-Webster Online, http://m-w.com/dictionary/tomography. Etymology: Greek *tomos* section + International Scientific Vocabulary *-graphy*.

for a proper interpretation. Therefore, the term "tomography" in relation to these techniques is a misnomer, which may lead to serious misunderstandings.

12.3 SELECTION OF STRUCTURES FOR LOCALIZATION

In spite of the mentioned problems, spatial localization of EEG sources is one of the most important issues that may lead to the renaissance of electroencephalography. Therefore, different EEG inverse solutions are being proposed in a multitude of studies, but the robustness of these algorithms is still far from the reliability of the true tomographies (CT, MRI, or PET). In the following we will not discuss differences between these algorithms, referring the reader to a rich literature on the topic.[3] Instead we will concentrate upon the sensitivity to noise present in the input data, which is common to all these solutions.

Inverse solutions have been mostly applied to instantaneous data (i.e., time points of the EEG data treated separately).[4] In the frequency domain, inverse solutions can be used as well due to the linearity of Fourier transform. However, given the complexity of the processes reflected in the brain's electrical activity, we cannot expect the distribution of current density in each time instant to fulfill the simplistic assumptions, like the minimum norm or maximum smoothness, used in computations of the EEG inverse solutions. Similarly, the configuration of sources contributing to a single frequency band is bound to change in time.

As suggested in the previous chapters (and many other studies), in most cases the best discrimination between EEG structures related to different processes can be achieved in the time-frequency plane. In Section 13.4 we presented additional advantages, offered by selective MP-based estimates, employing time-frequency definitions of relevant structures. In the following we will combine these advantages in a complete paradigm, using parameterization of relevant structures based upon multichannel matching pursuit as the input to the procedure computing an EEG inverse solution.

As presented in Section 8.2 and Figure 8.6, we can pool results of separate MP decompositions of EEG from several simultaneously recorded derivations. But, especially for tasks like the localization of cortical sources, we need a truly multichannel decomposition, finding similar waveforms simultaneously in all the channels. Some of the possible multichannel extensions of the matching pursuit

3 See [3, 7–11], and, for a review, see [12, 13].

4 Some advances have also been made to incorporate the temporal information for obtaining more reliable solutions [14, 15].

algorithm are described in Section 13.12. They differ with respect to the parameters of a single waveform, allowed to vary across the channels (obviously the amplitude, but potentially also phase or time position), and the criterion employed for choosing in each iteration the atom best matching the signals in all derivations at once (e.g., maximum sum of energies, sum of products, sum of moduli of products). In concordance with the model underlying instantaneous EEG inverse solutions, we choose the multichannel matching pursuit (MMP) with constant phases of the atoms fitted in all the channels. This basically relates to the algorithm MMP1, discussed in Section 13.12.

The major idea presented hereby relies on using amplitudes of the relevant structures, selected from the MMP expansion, as the input to an EEG inverse solution algorithm—in the following examples we use LORETA [3], which computes an instantaneous linear solution. LORETA implements a so-called distributed source model and so relies on reconstruction of the brain electric activity in each point of a 3-D grid of solution points, the number of points being much larger than the number of electrodes. Current densities estimated in each of these points constitute the solution. Slices of these 3-D images, referred to as "LORETA maps," are presented in Figures 12.1, 12.2 and Plate 8. Detailed discussion of the mathematical basis of this[5] or other EEG inverse solutions is beyond the scope of this book. The main point, which at the moment remains to be proved, is that the proposed paradigm should similarly improve the results of any other EEG/MEG inverse solution.

The process leading to the estimation of sources of selected structures is illustrated in Figure 12.1. From the MMP decomposition of multichannel EEG time series (presented in the upper left panel), we chose atoms conforming to the selected criteria—in this case sleep spindles. Time courses of the spindles found in the EEG epoch presented on the left are plotted in the upper right panel. We observe that—according to the constraints of the chosen MMP version—both structures have the same time courses across the channels, with different amplitudes. These amplitudes define the topography of structure intensities on the scalp electrodes. This topography, interpolated to the surface of the scalp, is presented in the leftmost lower panel. The same topography, confined to the values in the electrode positions, constitutes the input for the algorithm solving the EEG inverse problem. Its results

5 The implementation applied in this chapter's examples was developed in the Cuban Neuroscience Center, and uses a three concentric spheres model with solution space constrained to cortical gray matter and hippocampus (based upon the human brain atlas by [17]). The lead field was computed as defined by [18], and a LORETA algorithm [3] was used with an automatic setting of a regularization parameter based on the minimization of the generalized cross-validation function. The average Probabilistic MRI Atlas produced by the Montreal Neurological Institute [19–22] was used for computation and representation of the LORETA inverse solutions.

for both the spindles are presented in the slices on the right of the corresponding topographies.

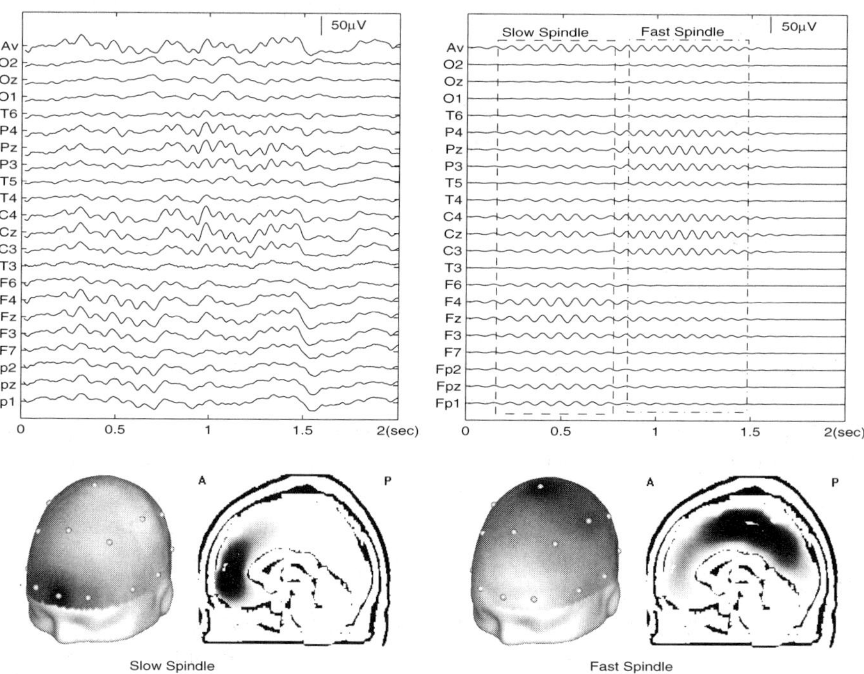

Figure 12.1 Upper left: 2 seconds of sleep EEG from 21 standard electrodes (uppermost trace—their average). Upper right: time courses of two Gabor functions (time-frequency atoms), conforming to the criteria assumed for sleep spindles, fitted to the EEG presented on the left by the multichannel matching pursuit. The first atom (slow spindle) is centered around 0.5 seconds and 11 Hz. Center of the second atom (fast spindle) is around 1 second and 14 Hz . Lower left: representation of the topographic signature of the slow spindle, pronounced in the frontal derivations, and the corresponding LORETA image. Lower right: the same for the fast spindle, pronounced in the parietal derivations. (Reprinted from [16], © 2005, with permission from Elsevier.)

12.4 LOCALIZATION OF SLEEP SPINDLES

In the first EEG study [16], a suboptimal version of the MMP was used for the sake of the speed of computations. It maximizes in each iteration the sum of products in all the channels. As discussed in Section 13.12, results of this algorithm (MMP2) are basically equivalent to MMP1, which maximizes the sum of energies rather than the sum of products.

MMP was applied to artifact-free epochs of sleep stage 2 from 20 overnight polysomnographic recordings, containing 21 EEG electrodes from the 10–20 system. From the resulting expansions, atoms corresponding to sleep spindles were automatically chosen based upon criteria corresponding to those described in Section 8.2, but the minimum amplitude of the sleep spindle was adjusted individually for each subject. As result, just like in the paradigm from Section 8.2, each of the detected sleep spindles was described in terms of time width, position, and frequency—but this time there was a different amplitude for each channel. These amplitudes defined, for each structure, a corresponding topography, defined by the distribution of amplitude across the electrodes. These topographies were used as the input for the LORETA inverse solution. This particular algorithm was chosen because of its popularity—it was used also in [23], a study we chose as a reference; using the same algorithm with different inputs facilitates a comparison of preprocessing schemes. A sample of results is given in Figure 12.2, presenting vertical slices of estimated current density for six sleep spindles, randomly chosen (one in each 0.5-Hz interval) from the few thousands of structures automatically detected in the analyzed polysomnographic recordings.

Details and discussion of these results can be found in [16]; hereby we discuss only the methodological conclusions stemming from the comparison with the reference study [23], based upon spectral integrals. In that case, 1.25-second-long epochs containing sleep spindles were carefully selected by visual analysis, together with reference EEG epochs containing no spindling activity. Subsequently, LORETA was used to estimate the 3-D intracerebral current density distribution for each frequency bin between 11.2 and 15.2 Hz. This corresponds to a visual selection of 1.25-second $\times$ 0.8-Hz boxes in the time-frequency plane, encompassing optimally the power of corresponding sleep spindles. However, the content of these boxes, which is due to the activity of sleep spindle generators, may at best statistically dominate other contributions. This effect, illustrated in Figure 11.1 and discussed in Chapter 11, is a direct consequence of the uncertainty principle in signal analysis [24].

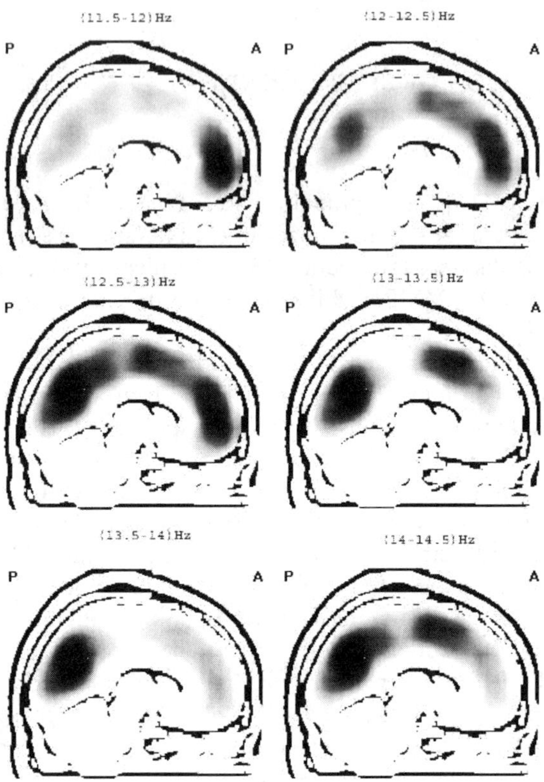

Figure 12.2 LORETA images calculated for six single sleep spindles, chosen at random from the frequency intervals from 11.5–12 Hz (top left) to 14–14.5 Hz (bottom right). In each of these ranges, chosen to correspond to the frequency bands used in [23], one spindle was randomly chosen from the structures automatically detected and parameterized via the MMP. Corresponding panels present LORETA images computed for these single sleep spindles. (Reprinted from [16], © 2005, with permission from Elsevier.)

Therefore, spectral integrals used as the input to inverse procedures also incorporate a large amount of unrelated activity, that is—in relation to the localization of the cortical generators of sleep spindles—noise. This noise was the reason why obtaining reasonable localizations in [23] required (a) careful visual selection of epochs containing sleep spindles, (b) statistical differentiation of LORETA images computed for these epochs with corresponding images for nonspindling EEG, and (c) pooling together (averaging) these results for hundreds of spindles, visually assigned to disjoint classes.

On the contrary, the MMP-based approach provided relatively clear LORETA images for *single* spindles (Figure 12.2), chosen automatically (that is via repeatable procedure), without any statistical postprocessing. This is mainly due to the selectivity of the matching pursuit estimates, discussed in Chapter 11.

Another application of this paradigm is presented in Plate 8. In that case localization was computed for atoms related to epileptic activity. MMP decomposition was performed according to algorithm MMP1, maximizing the sum of squares rather than the sum of products (MMP2). In this plate we observe that, contrary to Figure 12.1, waveforms in some of the channels have opposite phases (i.e., differ in the sign of the amplitude). In this case verification of results was provided by a presurgical electrocorticography (ECoG) of the same patient, which showed a broad area of epileptic discharges in locations corresponding to the area delineated by this procedure [25].

References

[1] J. Hadamard, *Lecture on the Cauchy Problem in Linear Partial Differential Equations*, New Haven, CT: Yale University Press, 1923.

[2] H. Helmholtz, "Über Einige Gesetze der Vertheilung Elektrischer Stroöme in Koörperlichen Leitern mit Anwendung auf die Thierisch-Elektrischen Versuche," *Ann Physik und Chemie*, vol. 9, 1853, pp. 211–33.

[3] R. D. Pascual-Marqui, C. M. Michel, and D. Lehman, "Low Resolution Electromagnetic Tomography: A New Method to Localize Electrical Activity in the Brain," *International Journal of Psychophysiology*, vol. 18, 1994, pp. 49–65.

[4] J. Z. Wang, S. J. Williamson, and L. Kaufman, "Magnetic Source Images Determined by a Leadfield Analysis—The Unique Minimum-Norm Least Squares Estimation," *IEEE Transactions on Biomedical Engineering*, vol. 39, 1992, pp. 231–251.

[5] M. S. Hämäläinen and R. J. Ilmoniemi, "Interpreting Magnetic Fields of the Brain: Minimum Norm Estimates," *Medical & Biological Engineering & Computing*, vol. 32, 1994, pp. 35–42.

[6] D. M. Schmidt, J. S. George, and C. C Wood, "Bayesian Inference Applied to the Biomagnetic Inverse Problem," *Human Brain Mapping*, vol. 7, 1999, pp. 195–212.

[7] N. J. Trujillo-Barreto, E. Aubert, and P. A. Valdés-Sosa, "Bayesian Model Averaging in EEG/MEG Imaging," *NeuroImage*, vol. 21, 2004, pp. 1300–1319.

[8] R. Grave de Peralta-Menendez and S. L. Gonzales-Andino, "Comparisons of Algorithms for the Localization of Focal Sources: Evaluation with Simulated Data and Analysis of Experimental Data," *International Journal of Bioelectromagnetism*, vol. 4, 2002, no. 1.

[9] R. Grave de Peralta-Menendez, et al., "Imaging the Electrical Activity of the Brain: ELECTRA," *Human Brain Mapping*, vol. 9, 2000, pp. 1–12.

[10] R. D. Pascual-Marqui, "Standardized Low-Resolution Brain Electromagnetic Tomography (sLORETA): Technical Details," *Methods & Findings in Experimental & Clinical Pharmacology*, vol. 24, 2002, pp. 5–12.

[11] J. Bosch-Bayard, et al., "3D Statistical Parametric Mapping of EEG Source Spectra by Means of Variable Resolution Electromagnetic Tomography (VARETA)," *Clinical Electroencephalography*, vol. 32, 2001, pp. 47–61.

[12] C. M. Michel, et al., "EEG Source Imaging," *Clinical Neurophysiology*, vol. 115, 2004, pp. 2195–2222.

[13] Z. J. Koles, "Trends in EEG Source Localization," *Electroencephalography and Clinical Neurophysiology*, vol. 106, 1998, pp. 127–137.

[14] O. Yamashita, et al., "Recursive Penalized Least Squares Solution for Dynamical Inverse Problems of EEG Generation," *Human Brain Mapping*, vol. 21, 2004, pp. 221–235.

[15] A. Galka, et al., "A Solution to the Dynamical Inverse Problem of EEG Generation Using Spatiotemporal Kalman Filtering," *NeuroImage*, vol. 23, 2004, pp. 435–453.

[16] P. J. Durka, et al., "Multichannel Matching Pursuit and EEG Inverse Solutions," *Journal of Neuroscience Methods*, vol. 148, no. 1, 2005, pp. 49–59.

[17] J. Talairach and P. Tournoux, *Co-Planar Stereotaxic Atlas of the Human Brain*, Stuttgart, 1988.

[18] J. Riera and M. E. Fuentes, "Electric Lead Field for a Piece-Wise Homogeneous Volume Conductor Model of the Head," *IEEE Transactions on Biomedical Engineering*, vol. 45, 1998, pp. 746–753.

[19] D. L. Collins, et al., "Automatic 3D Intersubject Registration of MR Volumetric in Standardized Talairach Space," *Journal of Computer Assisted Tomography*, vol. 18, 1994, pp. 192–205.

[20] A. C. Evans, et al., "3D Statistical Neuroanatomical Models from 305 MRI Volumes," *Proceedings of IEEE-Nuclear Science Symposium and Medical Imaging Conference*, vol. 95, 1993, pp. 1813–1817.

[21] A. C. Evans, et al., "Three-Dimensional Correlative Imaging: Applications in Human Brain Mapping," in *Functional Neuroimaging: Technical Foundations*, R. Thatcher, et al., (eds.), New York: Academic Press, 1994, pp. 145–161.

[22] J. C. Mazziotta, et al., "A Probabilistic Atlas of the Human Brain: Theory and Rationale for Its Development," *NeuroImage*, vol. 2, 1995, pp. 89–101.

[23] P. Anderer, et al., "Low-Resolution Brain Electromagnetic Tomography Revealed Simultaneously Active Frontal and Parietal Sleep Spindles Sources in the Human Cortex," *Neuroscience*, vol. 103, no. 3, 2001, pp. 581–592.

[24] S. Mallat, *A Wavelet Tour of Signal Processing*, 2nd ed., New York: Academic Press, 1999.

[25] A. Matysiak, et al., "Time-Frequency-Space Localization of Epileptic EEG Oscillations," *Acta Neurobiologiae Experimentalis*, vol. 65, 2005, pp. 435–442.

Part III

Equations and Technical Details

Chapter 13

Adaptive Approximations and Matching Pursuit

This chapter gives a mathematical description of adaptive time-frequency approximations and matching pursuit in time-frequency dictionaries.

Table 13.1

Symbols Used in the Following Chapters

$\langle x, y\rangle$	inner product of x and y: $\langle x, y\rangle = \int x(t)y^*(t)dt$
x^*	complex conjugate of x: $(a+bi)^* = a - bi$, where $i = \sqrt{-1}$
$\|\|x\|\|$	norm of the signal x; energy $\|\|x\|\|^2 = \langle x, x\rangle$
$\|a\|$	absolute value of number a
ω	angular frequency $\omega = \frac{2\pi}{T} = 2\pi f$

13.1 NOTATION

In the following sections, equations will be used for compact expression of ideas, rather than rigorous mathematical proofs—the latter can be found, for example, in [1]. Therefore, we use mostly formulae for continuous signals (that is, integrals rather than series), which are usually simpler and more elegant. Results obtained for continuous time functions can be viewed as asymptotic results for discrete sequences with sampling intervals decreasing to zero. These asymptotic results are precise enough to understand the behavior of discrete algorithms [1]. Table 13.1 lists mathematical symbols used in the following chapters.

13.2 LINEAR EXPANSIONS

To explore the unknown properties of signal $x(t)$, in the absence of a quantitative model of its generation, we may use a linear expansion in a set of known functions $\{g_1(t), g_2(t), \ldots, g_M(t)\}$:

$$x = \sum_{n=1}^{M} a_n g_n \tag{13.1}$$

If functions $\{g_n\}$ form an orthonormal basis, coefficients a_n are given simply by inner products of g_n with the signal:

$$a_n = \langle g_n, x\rangle = \int x(t) g_n^*(t) dt \tag{13.2}$$

Traditionally, orthogonal sets $\{g_n\}$ were limited to Dirac's deltas[1] δ_n and complex exponentials $e^{i\omega t}$, corresponding to the time-domain and spectral analyses. The first and most popular orthogonal wavelet bases are built from dilations and translations of a single function $\psi(\frac{t-u}{2^j})$. This implies the characteristic "zooming property" of wavelets (that is, increased time resolution and decreased frequency resolution at high frequencies). However, in the EEG analysis this often seems to be more of a drawback than an advantage. Only very special choices of the wavelet ψ give an orthogonal basis (see, for example, [1]). Actually, it was not before 1980 that the first such orthogonal sets were discovered. In recent decades, new orthogonal bases were found, like wavelet packets or local cosines.

To interpret (13.1), we relate those g_n that correspond to significant $|a_n|$ to the properties of the signal x. For example, large value of the product $\langle x, e^{i\omega_n t}\rangle$—a spectral peak at frequency ω_n—suggests that x contains periodic activity with base frequency near ω_n. However, presence of the same periodic activity may not be so evident if $|a_n|$ are calculated in a wavelet basis, since in this case energy will be diluted across several wavelets.

1 Discrete Dirac's delta is a sequence of zeros except for unity in the point i; that is, $\delta_i(k) = 1$ for $k = 1$ and zero otherwise.

13.3 TIME-FREQUENCY DISTRIBUTIONS

The most direct approach to estimation of signal's time-frequency energy density is the Wigner-Ville transform $\mathcal{W}$:

$$\mathcal{W}x = \int x\left(t + \frac{\tau}{2}\right) x^*\left(t - \frac{\tau}{2}\right) e^{-i\omega\tau} d\tau \tag{13.3}$$

However, as illustrated previously in Figure 4.9, it suffers from severe interferences, called cross-terms. Cross-terms are the area of a time-frequency energy density estimate that may be interpreted as indicating false presence of a signal's activity in given time and frequency coordinates. The problem of cross-terms was discussed in Section 4.4. Their origin can be deduced, for example, from (13.21).

Therefore, several reduced interference distributions (RID) were proposed to minimize this drawback. It can be achieved via the integration with kernel ϕ, which usually decreases the influence of cross-terms at a cost of lower time-frequency resolution. A general form of the Cohen's class of distributions (see [2, 3]) is given by

$$\mathcal{C}x = \int\int\int \phi(\theta,\tau) e^{-i(\theta t + \tau\omega - \theta u)} x\left(t + \frac{\tau}{2}\right) x^*\left(t - \frac{\tau}{2}\right) d\tau du d\theta \tag{13.4}$$

The most popular time-frequency distributions are spectrogram (squared modulus of the short-time Fourier transform) and scalogram (squared modulus of continuous wavelet transform). Similar to other time-frequency distributions, designed usually to minimize the cross-terms—and hence often termed reduced interference distributions (RID)—they can be derived from (13.4) with different kernels ϕ,[2] and they give better or worse results for different types of signals.

In general, to obtain a clear and robust picture of the time-frequency energy density for a given signal x, we must find an appropriate representation, tailored to the particular signal's content. However, there is no general recipe for this choice. Also, these quadratic representations do not offer a direct parameterization of a signal's features such as formula (13.1). Therefore, most of the techniques presented in this book, which work as filters in the space of parameters of functions fitted to the signal, cannot be used with quadratic time-frequency estimates of a signal's energy density.

2 To derive scalogram from (13.4), the kernel must change with frequency.

13.4 ADAPTIVE TIME-FREQUENCY APPROXIMATIONS

In the ideal situation we would like to have a linear expansion like (13.1), containing all those functions g_n that represent relevant structures of the signal x. Mere extension of the set $\{g_n\}$ beyond a basis does not solve the problem. Using large and redundant set of functions also increases the size of the representation and the difficulty of determination, which elements reflect important features of the signal. As illustrated in Figure 5.5, in a redundant set $\{g_n\}$—called a dictionary—many similar functions will give large values of inner products with the signal, so we would not know which of these functions should be actually treated as representative of the signal's features. Therefore, we must *choose* the functions $\{g_{\gamma_n}\}_{n=1\ldots M}$ adapted separately to represent the particular content of each analyzed signal. For a signal x of size N we seek an approximation in terms of M functions g_{γ_n} chosen from a redundant dictionary D:

$$x \approx \sum_{n=0}^{M-1} a_n g_{\gamma_n} \tag{13.5}$$

where $M \ll N \ll \text{size}(D)$. Criterion for choosing functions g_{γ_n} from D can be based upon minimal norm of the residue (that is, maximum variance explained by the expansion). In this context, we can define an optimal M-approximation as an expansion of the signal x by M functions chosen from dictionary D to minimize the following error ϵ:

$$\epsilon = \left\| x - \sum_{n=0}^{M-1} a_n g_{\gamma_n} \right\| \tag{13.6}$$

Unfortunately, finding such an optimal approximation is intractable, since the computational complexity of this problem grows exponentially with the dimension of the signal. In computer science such problems are termed "nonpolynomial" (i.e., of complexity growing with the size faster than any polynomial). Solving such problems, even for moderately sized input data, requires times easily exceeding the age of the universe.

The amount of computations needed to find an optimal expansion minimizing (13.6) is similar to what is needed for breaking advanced ciphers. It is so huge that we believe the ciphers to be safe. Actually, if we would find such optimal solution, it would also mean that we can break contemporary ciphers.[3] Therefore, we must rely on suboptimal solutions. The first efficient algorithm was proposed by Mallat and Zhang in 1993 in [6] under the name matching pursuit (a similar algorithm was also proposed in [7]).

13.5 MATCHING PURSUIT ALGORITHM

In the first step of the matching pursuit (MP), the waveform g_{γ_0} which best matches the signal x is chosen from dictionary D. In each of the consecutive steps, the waveform g_{γ_n} is matched to the signal $R^n x$, which is the residual left after subtracting results of previous iterations:

$$\begin{cases} R^0 x = x \\ R^n x = \langle R^n x, g_{\gamma_n} \rangle g_{\gamma_n} + R^{n+1} x \\ g_{\gamma_n} = \arg\max_{g_{\gamma_i} \in D} |\langle R^n x, g_{\gamma_i} \rangle| \end{cases} \tag{13.7}$$

For very large—or potentially infinite—dictionaries, it may not be possible to find in each iteration the function g_γ that exactly satisfies the condition in the last line of (13.7), giving the largest product with the residuum. Fortunately, if we manage to find in each iteration a function g_{γ_n} that best fits the signal up to an

3 We can formulate an almost equivalent decision problem, asking whether for a given dictionary of functions $D = \{g_\gamma\}$, $\epsilon_1 > 0$, and signal x exists an M-approximation giving error (13.6) smaller than ϵ_1. It can be proved [4] to belong to the NP-complete class of problems possessing the two following properties [5]:

- Finding a solution requires exponential (nonpolynomial) time, but given solution can be checked in polynomial (P) time. The name "nondeterministic-polynomial" (NP) stems from the lack of a deterministic algorithm finding this answer in polynomial time ("guessing" the right answer is nondeterministic).
- The solution to each of the problems from the NP-class can be translated into solution of any other problem from this class in a polynomial time.

This class encompasses a variety of important problems, from the classical traveling salesman problem to factorization of large numbers, which has direct implications in cryptography. In particular, strength of the public key cryptography depends on factorization. Therefore, if for any problem from the NP class, a polynomial-time solution is found, it can be used to break the contemporary public key cryptography. Nevertheless, we are still using this system for securing transmission of sensitive data (e.g., credit card numbers) over the Internet. It is generally believed that NP-complete problems do not have polynomial-time solutions, yet this basic theorem (P≠NP) is still not proved—it may be also undecidable from the currently applied axioms.

optimality factor α, that is

$$|\langle x, g_{\gamma_n}\rangle| \geq \alpha \sup_{g_\gamma \in D} |\langle x, g_\gamma\rangle| \tag{13.8}$$

then (13.7) still can be proved[4] to converge to x, that is

$$x = \sum_{n=0}^{+\infty} \langle R^n x,\ g_{\gamma_n}\rangle g_{\gamma_n} \tag{13.9}$$

In practice we use finite expansions:

$$x = \sum_{n=0}^{M-1} \langle R^n x,\ g_{\gamma_n}\rangle g_{\gamma_n} + R^M x \tag{13.10}$$

or, equivalently,

$$x \approx \sum_{n=0}^{M-1} \langle R^n x,\ g_{\gamma_n}\rangle g_{\gamma_n} \tag{13.11}$$

The number M in this expansion equals the number of iterations of (13.7). Therefore, the choice of M is referred to as the stopping criterion; it will be discussed in Section 13.7.

Although the functions g_γ from a redundant dictionary are not orthogonal, each residuum $R^{n+1}x$ is by construction orthogonal to the function g_{γ_n} chosen in a given iteration, which implies energy conservation:

$$||x||^2 = \sum_{n=0}^{M-1} |\langle R^n x,\ g_{\gamma_n}\rangle|^2 + ||R^m x||^2 \tag{13.12}$$

13.6 ORTHOGONALIZATION

In Section 9.2 we discussed the suboptimality of the greedy MP algorithm. Neither the weights nor the selected functions are exactly optimal in the sense of minimizing error (13.6). Although, as stated in the previous section, the optimal solution is

4 If the dictionary D is complete, which is the case for any dictionary containing a basis. For the proof of convergence, see [6].

intractable, there are several possibilities to improve the representation and decrease its error for a given M (13.10).

A posteriori adjustment of the weights of the chosen functions, proposed in [6], relies on projection of the signal onto the space spanned by these functions. Such a post-orthogonalization or back-projection requires inversion of large matrices or the use of some iterative descent method. Orthogonalization can also be performed after each step of (13.7) to minimize the possibility of readmission of a previously chosen function; this approach was called orthogonal matching pursuit [8]. It can be achieved either by adjusting the weights of the original dictionary's functions or via orthogonalization of the chosen functions. Finally, instead of orthogonalizing the sets of functions chosen by the standard procedure, we can choose the best of orthogonalized functions. This approach requires orthogonalization of the entire dictionary to the set of functions accumulated in each iteration.

These variants give improvements in convergence, which are significant mostly for higher iterations, since the functions chosen in early iterations are usually almost orthogonal anyway. Of course, in the rate distortion sense—that is, the amount of energy explained in a given number of iterations—these algorithms will never give worse results than the standard MP. Gains offered by these procedures may justify the increase of computational expenses in applications like compression, when the relative error achieved for given M is the most important variable to be minimized and retaining a small dictionary size is beneficial if we store/transmit the indices of dictionary's functions instead of their exact parameters. However, for the kind of applications presented in this book, increasing the size (that is, density) of the dictionary looks like a more reasonable (than orthogonalization) use of computing resources, as it offers direct gains in terms of accuracy of parameterization of particular signal structures[5] or the overall robustness of the time-frequency estimate of energy density. However, a direct comparison of different variants of the MP algorithm in this respect was not presented up to now.

13.7 STOPPING CRITERIA

A stopping criterion regulates the number of waveforms M included in MP expansion (13.11). Different criteria were briefly discussed in Section 9.4. Let us

5 Most of the waveforms analyzed in Chapter 8 were fitted in relatively early iterations of MP, where the differences between the standard and orthogonalized versions of the algorithms are rather small, since, as we mentioned, most of the functions chosen in early iterations are nearly orthogonal anyway.

recall that the simplest one, relatively robust in routine applications, simply fixes a priori the number of iterations M, irrelevant of the content of the analyzed signal. Application of this criterion in practice requires a solid prior experience with decompositions of signals of a given length and particular characteristics.

Another simple criterion can be based upon the percentage of a signal's energy, explained by the MP expansion: we stop the decomposition (13.7) when the energy of expansion (13.11), $\sum_{n=0}^{M-1} |\langle R^n x,\ g_{\gamma_n}\rangle|^2$, reaches a given percentage of the signal's energy $||x||^2$, say 99%. Although an energetic criterion at a first glance looks physically plausible, the actual results of decompositions based upon this criterion can be dramatically impaired in cases when a few high-energy structures—which can be due to a linear trend, DC offset, or low-frequency artifacts—may saturate the chosen percentage before even reaching the actual information content of the signal.

We can also stop the decomposition when $|\langle R^n x,\ g_{\gamma_n}\rangle|^2$ (that is, the energy of the function added in the last iteration) reaches a certain threshold. It can be seen as the achieved energy resolution of the representation (13.11). It may be an optimal choice for achieving uniform resolutions for the decomposition of smaller parts of a larger signal [9] or image [10, 11]. However, the value of this threshold has to be decided a priori. An example application of this criterion is given in Section 9.4.

A stopping criterion, which takes into account the information content of the signal, was proposed in [6]. It relies on the idea of decomposing only the part of the signal that is coherent with the applied dictionary. Correlation of the signal x with dictionary D can be defined as

$$\lambda(x) = \sup_{g_\gamma \in D} \frac{|\langle x, g_\gamma\rangle|}{||x||} \tag{13.13}$$

We notice that this correlation is equal to the relative energy explained by the algorithm (13.7) in the first iteration.[6] Similarly, we can define the correlation of the n-th residuum with the dictionary as

$$\lambda(R^n x) = \sup_{g_\gamma \in D} \frac{|\langle R^n x, g_\gamma\rangle|}{||R^n x||} \tag{13.14}$$

Again, in terms of the MP algorithm (13.7), this reflects the percentage of the energy of the residuum, explained in the nth iteration. When this correlation drops

6 For the sake of simplicity we omit here details related to the local search of the neighborhood of γ in each step. A complete formal treatment of this issue can be found in [6].

below a certain threshold, it may indicate that the decomposed signal (that is its nth residuum) is no longer coherent with the dictionary, and further iterations will not contribute information on its structure. Such a signal can be understood as noise with respect to the applied dictionary;[7] for the Gabor dictionary (discussed in the next section), it is a white noise process. When decomposing white noise in the Gabor dictionary, $\lambda(R^n x)$ quickly reaches an asymptotic value λ_N^∞, which depends on the size of the signal N. If we estimate (e.g., by numerical experiments) λ_N^∞, we can estimate $\lambda(R^n x)$ in each step of (13.7) and stop the decomposition of a signal of size N when

$$\lambda(R^n x) > \lambda_N^\infty \tag{13.15}$$

13.8 MATCHING PURSUIT WITH GABOR DICTIONARIES

Real-valued Gabor function can be expressed as

$$g_\gamma(t) = K(\gamma) e^{-\pi\left(\frac{t-u}{s}\right)^2} \cos\left(\omega(t-u)+\phi\right), \tag{13.16}$$

where $K(\gamma)$ is such that $||g_\gamma|| = 1$. These functions provide a general and compact model for transient oscillations; also, (13.16) can describe parametrically a wide variety of shapes, as presented in Figure 5.2. Finally, Gabor functions exhibit good (i.e., relatively compact) time-frequency localization [1]. Gabor dictionaries were used in all the studies presented in this book. However, dictionaries composed from other types of functions can be also used with the MP algorithm (13.7); for example, an efficient implementation of MP with dictionaries of damped sinusoids was presented in [12].

Parameters $\Gamma = (u, \omega, s)$ from (13.16) constitute a three-dimensional[8] continuous space, yielding a potentially infinite size of a Gabor dictionary D_∞. Even if we discretize the parameters of the Gabor functions, which can be reasonably[9] fitted to the signal of given length N, we get a huge number of candidate functions (of the order of N^3). For example, for $N = 1{,}000$ points (that is, at best few seconds of EEG) and unit discretization steps $u = 1 \ldots N$, $s = 1 \ldots N$ and

7 The notion of noise in signal processing is not well defined. Usually, it is understood as the information that cannot be understood within the applied framework.

8 Phase ϕ is optimized separately in practical implementations—see Section 14.1.

9 Numerically, to a signal of length N we may fit any Gabor. But in practice we limit the dictionaries to functions that may reasonably explain the structures contained in the signal—usually, widths s not exceeding the signal length, time centers u within the signal boundaries, and frequencies ω below the Nyquist frequency.

$\omega = (1 \ldots N)\pi/N$, we get 10^9 functions. It is not feasible to search such a huge space in each iteration of (13.7).

For the actual implementations of MP with Gabor dictionaries, we carefully select a subset D_a of the potentially infinite dictionary D_∞, and the choice of g_{γ_n} in each iteration is performed in two steps. First we perform a complete search of the subset D_a to find parameters $\tilde{\gamma}$ of a function $g_{\tilde{\gamma}}$, giving the largest product with the residuum

$$\tilde{\gamma} = \arg \max_{g_\gamma \in D_a} |\langle R^n x, g_\gamma \rangle| \tag{13.17}$$

and then we search the neighborhood of the parameters $\tilde{\gamma}$ for a function g_{γ_n}, giving possibly an even larger product $\langle R^n x, g_{\gamma_n} \rangle$ than $\langle R^n x, g_{\tilde{\gamma}} \rangle$. This local search can be implemented either by a complete search—corresponding to (13.7)—in a dense subdictionary, constructed for an appropriately chosen neighborhood of $\tilde{\gamma}$ as in [13], or via significantly faster Newton gradient search as in [6], which, however, can end up in a local minimum.

In any case, there is no guarantee that this refinement will improve the fit, since $\tilde{\gamma}$ can be a local maximum. Therefore, as the worst case we must take the scenario when the local search does not improve the results, which corresponds to performing plain MP given by (13.7) in the dictionary D_a only. This fact stresses the importance of the choice of D_a. The first recipe for this choice is based upon the following theorem, proved in [6]:

If we choose basic intervals for time and frequency such that

$$\Delta u = \frac{\Delta \omega}{2\pi} < 1 \tag{13.18}$$

and a dilation factor $a > 1$, and construct a subdictionary D_a from the functions g_γ with parameters $\gamma = (u, \omega, s)$ chosen as

$$\gamma = \left(p\, a^j \Delta u,\ k \frac{\Delta \omega}{a^j},\ a^j \right) \tag{13.19}$$

for integer j, k, p, then for any signal $x \in \mathbf{L}^2(\mathbf{R})$, where $\mathbf{L}^2(\mathbf{R})$ is the Hilbert space of square-integrable functions (that is, functions of finite energy) there exists an optimality factor $\alpha > 0$ such that

$$\sup_{g_\gamma \in D_a} |\langle x, g_\gamma \rangle| \geq \alpha \sup_{g_\gamma \in D_\infty} |\langle x, g_\gamma \rangle| \tag{13.20}$$

Optimality factor α relates to the maximum relative loss in accuracy—measured in terms of energy explained in a single iteration—stemming from operating on a particular discrete subset D_a of a continuous Gabor dictionary D. If D_a

is chosen according to (13.19), we know that $\alpha > 0$, but no other estimates for α can be found for a particular D_a—they all depend on the signal x. Also, the choice of the time and frequency intervals Δu and $\Delta\omega$, and the scale parameter a, is still somehow arbitrary. We know only that smaller values of these parameters result in larger dictionaries D_a, and hence potentially better MP decompositions.

To find an optimal relation between sampling of the time/frequency and scale parameters, we may construct D_a from uniformly spaced Gabor functions. However, for this purpose we must apply a metrics relevant to the MP decomposition, related to the inner product between the g_{γ_1} and g_{γ_2}, rather than the distance between the sets of parameters γ_1 and γ_2. Such work, leading to an optimal sampling of Gabor dictionaries governed by a single density parameter, and an accountable measure of a single-iteration error of MP, is currently in progress [14].

13.9 STATISTICAL BIAS

Matching pursuit in structured dictionaries, constructed according to fixed schemes like (13.19), is likely to introduce a statistical bias in the resulting decomposition. Statistical properties of the decomposition are significant only for analysis of large amounts of data, but in such cases—as will be presented later—they may lead to methodological artifacts and erroneous conclusions.

Figure 13.1 compares MP decompositions of the same data (sample EEG and simulated noise) in two different dictionaries. The left column presents results obtained by MP with the dyadic dictionary, constructed according to (13.19) as proposed in [6]. The right column gives results obtained with stochastic dictionaries [15], which are a priori free from any fixed structure—parameters of functions were drawn from flat distributions before each decomposition.

In decompositions performed using the dyadic dictionary (left column), even for the white noise (upper and middle rows) we observe a repetitive structure, which is actually absent in the decomposed data (noise). It is a methodological artifact, related to the structure of the dictionary employed in MP decomposition. This structure is absent in the right column, where results of noise decomposition in stochastic dictionaries reveal the expected uniform distribution of parameters in the time-frequency plane (peak in the middle of frequency range results from the convention of assigning half of the Nyquist frequency to Dirac's deltas). The same stands for decompositions of real EEG data (50 epochs, bottom row): while the right histogram of frequencies from decompositions in the stochastic dictionary corresponds well to the classical EEG spectrum, in the left histogram from dyadic

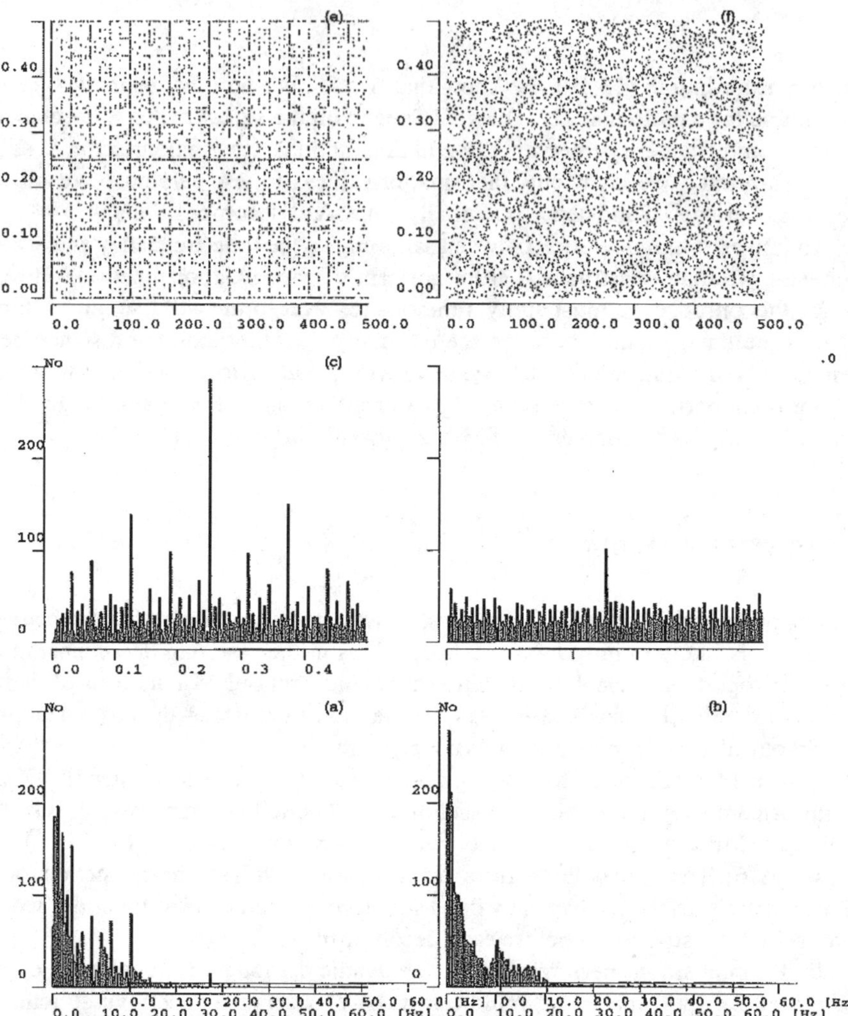

Figure 13.1 MP decompositions of the same signals in dyadic (right column) and stochastic (left column) dictionaries. Upper and middle row—time-frequency centers (upper) and histograms of frequencies (middle) of functions fitted to white noise. Bottom row—histograms of frequency centers of functions fitted to EEG. The peak in the middle of the frequency range, present in the middle right panel, results from the convention of assigning half of Nyquist frequency to Dirac's deltas, frequently fitted to noise. (Reprinted from [16] with permission. © 2001 by PTBUN and IBD.)

decompositions we may erroneously detect some resonant frequencies—again a methodological error, as a property of the procedure rather than analyzed data. Unbiased representations in these figures—and in most of the studies presented in this book—were obtained using the MP implementation described in [15], which relies on drawing the parameters (u, ω, s) of the dictionary's functions from flat probability distributions. Alternatively, statistical bias can be avoided by a proper randomization of the parameters initially chosen from other than flat distributions.

If statistical properties of the decomposition are important, such randomization should be performed before decomposition of each subsequent data epoch. However, statistical bias as such does not impair the *quality* of the representation (e.g., in the distortion rate sense). This issue must be taken into account only when pooling results of decompositions of large amounts of data.

13.10 MP-BASED ESTIMATE OF SIGNAL'S ENERGY DENSITY

Calculating the Wigner distribution of expansion (13.11) would yield

$$\mathcal{W}x \approx \mathcal{W}\left(\sum_{n=0}^{M-1} a_n g_{\gamma_n}\right) = \sum_{n=0}^{M-1} a_n^2 \, \mathcal{W}g_{\gamma_n} + \sum_{n=0}^{M-1} \sum_{k=1, k\neq n}^{M-1} a_n a_k^* \, \mathcal{W}\left(g_{\gamma_n}, g_{\gamma_k}\right) \tag{13.21}$$

where $a_n = \langle R^n x, \ g_{\gamma_n} \rangle$, and $\mathcal{W}\left(g_{\gamma_n}, g_{\gamma_k}\right)$ is a cross-Wigner transform of g_{γ_n} and g_{γ_k} given by

$$\mathcal{W}\left(g_{\gamma_n}, g_{\gamma_k}\right) = \int g_{\gamma_n}\left(t + \frac{\tau}{2}\right) g_{\gamma_k}^*\left(t - \frac{\tau}{2}\right) e^{-i\omega\tau} d\tau \tag{13.22}$$

The double sum in (13.21) contains the cross-terms. Due to the representation (13.11), we can omit them explicitly and construct the time-frequency representation of signal's energy density from the first sum, containing auto-terms:

$$\mathcal{E}x = \sum_{n=0}^{M-1} a_n^2 \, \mathcal{W}g_{\gamma_n} \tag{13.23}$$

Energy conservation of this distribution is easily demonstrated (see [6]).

The idea of stochastic dictionaries can be also applied to improve time-frequency representation of energy of a single data epoch. Let's consider a signal, presented in Figure 13.2, simulated according to (13.24):

$$x(t) = \begin{cases} \sin\left(0.625\pi t \sin(0.002\pi t)\right), & t = 0 \ldots 299 \\ \sin\left(0.007(t-300)^2\right), & t = 300 \ldots 512 \end{cases} \tag{13.24}$$

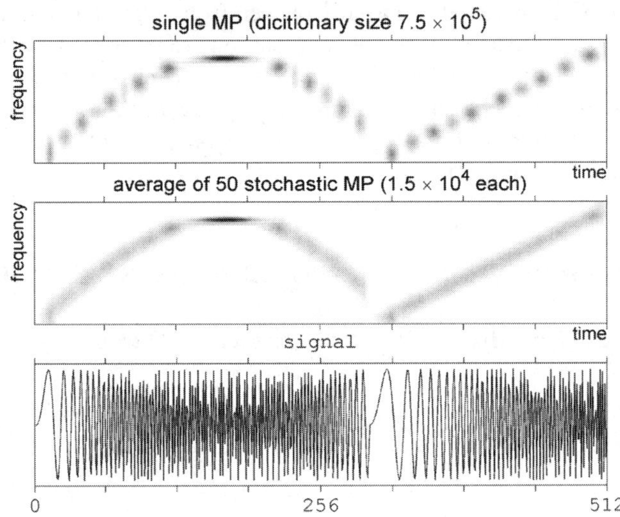

Figure 13.2 Energy density $\mathcal{E}x(t,\omega)$ from (13.23), proportional to shades of gray, of a simulated signal [bottom plot, (13.24)] calculated from single MP decomposition over a dictionary containing 7.5×10^5 waveforms (top) and averaged over 50 decompositions in different realizations of stochastic dictionaries, containing 1.5×10^4 atoms each (middle plot). (*From:* [15]. © 2001 IEEE. Reprinted with permission.)

The upper plot of Figure 13.2 presents the result of decomposition of this signal over a large dictionary (7.5×10^5 Gabor functions). In spite of the high resolution of this decomposition, the changing frequency is represented by a series of structures, since all the dictionary's functions have constant frequency. The middle plot of Figure 13.2 shows an average of 50 time-frequency representations constructed from decompositions over different realizations of small (1.5×10^4) stochastic dictionaries. Their size was optimized for representation of this particular signal, and the number of averaged decompositions was chosen to make the computational costs of both representations equal. The plot in the middle panel corresponds better to (13.24). However, it is constructed from 50 times more waveforms than the upper plot, so the underlying parameterization is not compact.

13.11 AN INTERESTING FAILURE OF THE GREEDY ALGORITHM

Suboptimal solution of an intractable problem (Section 13.4) must have its price. Mathematical examples of failures in pattern recognition, due to the greedy strategy (13.7) applied by the matching pursuit, were presented in [17, 18]. In the following, we present and discuss an example referring directly to the transient oscillatory activity relevant to the content of EEG.

Signal (R^0) in Figure 13.3 is composed from two Gabor functions, both of them actually present in the dictionary D_a used for the decomposition (Section 13.8). In spite of that, we observe (in the right column) that the first function (g_0), fitted to the signal, is completely different from either of the two functions from which the signal was composed! According to (13.7), the MP algorithm has chosen the function g_0 giving the largest product $\langle x, g_0 \rangle$ in a *single* step. Of course, taking into account the next steps, this decision was definitely not optimal. Choosing the two Gabors, which were exactly represented in D_a, would explain 100% of signal's energy in only two iterations. However, as a consequence of the first choice, the following residues (left column of Figure 13.3) must be explained by several different Gabor functions.

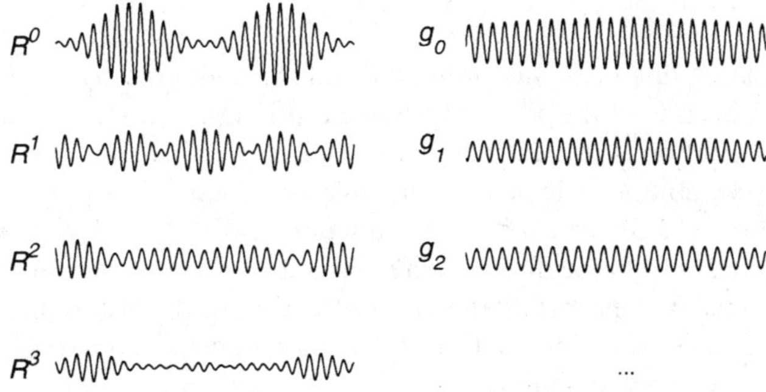

Figure 13.3 A failure in feature extraction: R^0—analyzed signal (upper left), g_0—function fitted in the first iteration by the MP algorithm (upper right). Horizontal—time, vertical—amplitude, both in arbitrary units (simulated signal). The left column presents subsequent residues left after subtracting functions fitted in corresponding iterations presented in the right column.

Such an effect occurs only if both Gabors present in the signal have not only the same frequencies, but also the same phase. Such a coincidence is likely to occur in a biological signal only if both the structures are produced by the same generator. And still, MP represents them jointly only if their time centers are close enough. Larger displacement of these structures would result in separate representation even in such a synchronized case. Therefore, we may argue that this effect, mathematically classified as a failure of the suboptimal procedure, is actually a welcome feature in the analysis of physiological signals. It was already presented on epileptic EEG in Section 9.2, where interpretation in terms of a certain measure of periodicity was proposed.

Some of similar "failures" of the matching pursuit (see [17, 18]) can be properly resolved by orthogonalized versions of MP, discussed in Section 13.5. We can also modify the similarity function (criterion) used in each step of (13.7) to choose the "best fit." High resolution pursuit, proposed in [19], is a variant of the MP procedure; it relies on an arbitrary parameter regulating the balance between the local and global fits. Its version, tailored for exact representation of sounds with sharp attack and relatively slow decay, was presented in [20]; it resulted in increased time resolution at a cost of frequency resolution.

Finally, representations optimal in the sense of the sparseness can be achieved via global minimization of the ℓ^1 norm of the representation's coefficients—that is,

$$\sum_{n=0}^{M-1} |a_n| = \min$$

Implementation of this idea was presented in [18] under the name Basis Pursuit. Unfortunately, in spite of the advances in linear programming, computational complexity of this solution is still extremely high for reasonably sized problems.

If we were able to calculate in practice an optimal M-approximation (i.e., minimizing error (13.6) for a set of M functions g_{γ_n}), these functions would be potentially different from the first M in an optimal $M+1$-approximation, computed for the same signal in the same dictionary. With the iterative MP solution (13.7), the choice of the first M functions does not depend on how many waveforms in total are included in the representation.

13.12 MULTICHANNEL MATCHING PURSUIT

Contrary to the relatively well-defined monochannel case, the term "multichannel matching pursuit" (MMP)—even if restricted to the time-frequency dictionaries of Gabor functions—can refer to one of several, significantly different, approaches. Differences between MMP algorithms can be mostly attributed to the two following groups of settings:

A. Structure of the multichannel dictionary (i.e., which parameters of the time-frequency atoms are allowed to vary across the channels);

B. Criterion used for choosing (in each iteration) the atom, best fitting the residua in all the channels simultaneously.

Different settings of these conditions result in different properties of resulting algorithms and multichannel decompositions. Starting from the most straightforward setup described in the next section, we may relax constraints in (A), allowing, for example, for different phases (MMP3), or different time centers,[10] of the atoms fitted in different channels. The criterion (B), minimized in each step of MMP, can be varied to allow for a computational optimization, as in [22], or to impose some additional, model-based prior constraints on the solution, as in [23]. Obviously, there are several possible combinations of these conditions, which can be adjusted for particular tasks. We shall discuss only a few examples, possibly relevant to the analysis of EEG/MEG. Enumerative names for some of the variations of MMP, introduced in the following subsections, were assigned for referencing within this book.

MMP1: Constant Phase, Maximum Sum of Energies

The most straightforward multichannel extension of the MP—let's call it MMP1—can be defined by the following conditions [24]:

A1. Only the amplitude varies across channels.

B1. We maximize the sum of squared products (energies) in all the channels.

Let us denote the multichannel signal as $\mathbf{x}$, and the signal in the ith channel as $\mathbf{x}^i$, with $i = 1 \ldots N_c$, where N_c is the number of channels. We may express the condition (B1) for the choice of atom g_γ in n-th iteration as

$$\max_{g_\gamma \in D} \sum_{i=1}^{N_c} |\langle R^n \mathbf{x}^i, g_\gamma \rangle|^2 \tag{13.25}$$

10 This approach was implemented in an algorithm designed for decomposition of stereo sound signals, by introducing a time delay between channels [21].

The whole procedure can be described as

$$\begin{cases} R^0\mathbf{x} = \mathbf{x} \\ R^n\mathbf{x}^i = \langle R^n\mathbf{x}^i, g_{\gamma_n}\rangle g_{\gamma_n} + R^{n+1}\mathbf{x}^i \\ g_{\gamma_n} = \arg\max_{g_\gamma \in D} \sum_{i=1}^{N_c} |\langle R^n\mathbf{x}^i, g_\gamma\rangle|^2 \end{cases} \tag{13.26}$$

Results of MMP1 are given in terms of functions g_{γ_n}, selected in consecutive iterations, and their weights in all the channels, determined for channel i by the real-valued products $\langle R^n\mathbf{x}^i, g_{\gamma_n}\rangle$. In each iteration, the multichannel residuum $R^{n+1}\mathbf{x}$ is computed by subtracting from the previous residua in each channel i the contribution of g_{γ_n}, weighted by $\langle R^n\mathbf{x}^i, g_{\gamma_n}\rangle$.

MMP2: Constant Phase, Maximum Sum of Products

Assumption of invariant phase in all the channels was explored in [22] (Section 12.4) to yield an efficient decomposition algorithm. If we modify the criterion of choice from the previous section to

$$\max_{g_\gamma \in D} \left| \sum_{i=1}^{N_c} \langle R^n\mathbf{x}^i, g_\gamma\rangle \right|, \tag{13.27}$$

we get the conditions:

A2. Only the amplitude varies across the channels.

B2. We maximize the absolute value of the sum of products across channels.

Due to the linearity of the residuum operator R [22], this choice allows for implementing a simple trick. Instead of finding in each step the product of each dictionary's waveform with all the channels separately, and then computing their sum (13.27), in each step we decompose the average signal $\bar{\mathbf{x}}$

$$\bar{\mathbf{x}} = \frac{1}{N_c} \sum_{i=1}^{N_c} \mathbf{x}^i \tag{13.28}$$

$$\begin{cases} R^0\bar{\mathbf{x}} = \bar{\mathbf{x}} \\ R^n\bar{\mathbf{x}} = \langle R^n\bar{\mathbf{x}}, g_{\gamma_n}\rangle g_{\gamma_n} + R^{n+1}\bar{\mathbf{x}} \\ \mathbf{g}_{\gamma_n} = \arg\max_{\mathbf{g}_\gamma \in D} |\langle R^n\bar{\mathbf{x}}, g_\gamma\rangle| \\ R^n\mathbf{x}^i = \langle R^n\mathbf{x}^i, g_{\gamma_n}\rangle g_{\gamma_n} + R^{n+1}\mathbf{x}^i \end{cases} \tag{13.29}$$

This procedure yields a computational complexity close to the monochannel MP—compared to MMP3, reduced by the factor N_c (that is, number of channels). Convergence of this procedure may be relatively slower for waveforms appearing in different channels with exactly opposite phases. If weights of such a structure cause its *total and exact* cancellation in the average signal $R^n\bar{\mathbf{x}}$, as simulated in Figure 13.4, it may even be completely omitted in the expansion computed by MMP2. Nevertheless, if this cancellation is not complete, and a trace of the atom g_{γ_n} is still present in $R^n\bar{\mathbf{x}}$, then it should be correctly parameterized by the products $\langle R^n\mathbf{x}^i, \mathbf{g}_{\gamma_n}\rangle$—probably in a later iteration as compared to MMP1.

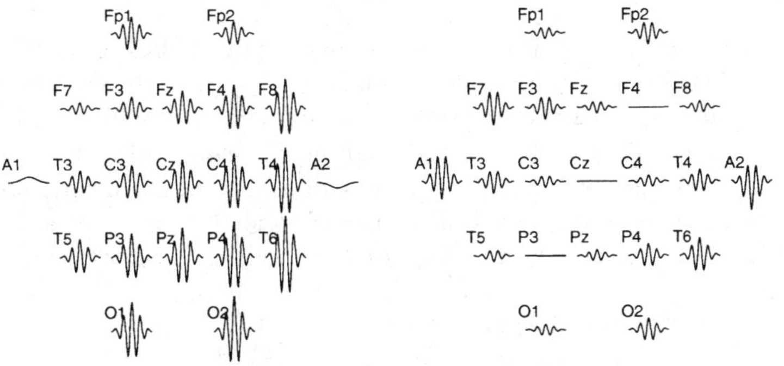

Figure 13.4 Simulated example of the same EEG waveform, presented in reference to linked ears (A1+A2, left panel) and to a central Cz (right panel). We observe that Cz reference introduces structures in opposite phases in derivations from left/frontal and right/parietal locations. (Reprinted from [22] with permission. © 2005 by PTBUN and IBD.)

Due to operating on the average of channels, this version of the algorithm cannot be directly applied to the data presented in the average reference. This problem is absent in MMP1 as well as in the next implementation, allowing for arbitrary phases across the channels.

MMP3: Variable Phase, Maximum Sum of Energies

A3. Phase and amplitude vary across the channels.

B3. We maximize the sum of squared products (energies) across channels.

Again, as in (13.25), we maximize

$$\max_{g_\gamma \in D} \sum_{i=1}^{N_c} |\langle R^n \mathbf{x}^i, g_\gamma^i \rangle|^2 \tag{13.30}$$

but this time $g_{\gamma_n}^i$ are not the same g_{γ_n} for all channels i—they can have different phases.

$$\begin{cases} R^0 \mathbf{x} = \mathbf{x} \\ R^n \mathbf{x}^i = \langle R^n \mathbf{x}^i, g_{\gamma_n}^i \rangle g_{\gamma_n}^i + R^{n+1} \mathbf{x}^i \\ g_{\gamma_n} = \arg \max_{\mathbf{g}_\gamma \in D} \sum_{i=1}^{N_c} |\langle R^n \mathbf{x}^i, g_\gamma^i \rangle|^2 \end{cases} \tag{13.31}$$

As presented in Section 14.1, computing an optimal phase of Gabor function g_γ, maximizing absolute value of the product $\langle R^n \mathbf{x}^i, g_\gamma \rangle$, can be implemented very efficiently. Value of (13.25) for phases optimized separately will never be smaller than in the case of the phase common to all the channels, so this freedom should improve the convergence. Equivalently, phase of g_γ can be also incorporated in the complex weights in each channel, if we use complex Gabor atoms and calculate their products with the Hilbert transform of a real-valued signal $\mathbf{x}$ (see [25]).

Other MMP Variants and Applications

By applying different combinations of the interchannel constraints on parameters (A) and criteria of choice (B), we can construct an arbitrary number of different MMP decompositions. Ideally, these constraints and criteria should reflect the assumed model of generation of the underlying multichannel signals. For example, MMP tailored for the analysis of stereo recordings of sound in [21] allows for different time positions of the time-frequency atoms present in the two channels. Together with different amplitudes in each channel, it relates to modeling the microphones as gain-delay filters in the anechoic case. Unfortunately, a model explaining relations between channels of EEG/MEG recordings is far more complicated, even in the case of known distribution of sources (so-called forward EEG problem). Characteristics of sources contributing to given signal structures are not known a priori, which leads to the ill-posed inverse EEG problem (Section 12.1).

An attempt to incorporate constraints, reflecting the generation of multichannel EEG, into the MMP procedure, was presented in [23]. To the purely energetic criterion of MMP1 (13.25), a second term was added to favor those g_γ which give smooth distribution of amplitudes across the channels. Spatial smoothness (quantified by Laplacian operators) means basically that the values of $\langle R^n \mathbf{x}^i, g_\gamma \rangle$ should be similar for i corresponding to the neighboring channels. However, a choice combining two completely different criteria requires some setting of their relative weights. For example, if we attribute too much importance to the spatial criterion, in favor of the energetic one, we may obtain atoms giving very smooth scalp distributions across electrodes. But in such a case the convergence of the MMP procedure, measured in the rate-distortion sense, relating to the amount of explained energy, may be severely impaired. Up to now, no objective or optimal settings for regulating the influence of such extra criteria on the MMP algorithms was proposed. Therefore, all the applications of MMP presented in this book (Chapter 12) are based upon the relatively well-understood and free of arbitrary settings procedures (MMP2 and MMP3).

A procedure that is free of task-specific settings also has obvious advantages stemming directly from its generality. For example, exactly the same algorithm (MMP3) that was used in [22] for parameterization of the epileptic EEG in subsequent channels can be applied to decomposing subsequent trials of event-related potentials. One can also envisage instantaneous decomposition of both repetitions and channels of event-related potentials, with some of the discussed constraints applied separately to the relevant dimensions.

This might result in improved properties of the ERD/ERS estimates, compared to the estimation based upon separate MP decompositions as presented in Chapter 10. Apart from that, it may be also used to compute estimates of the phase locking factor [26] (also called intertrial coherence, [27]). Simultaneous decomposition of all the repetitions will be crucial in this case: in separate MP decompositions of subsequent trials, atoms representing possibly the same structures can have slightly different frequencies, which makes their relative phase insignificant.

Finally, before allowing for variations of any of the other parameters, we must also consider—apart from the potential value of such models—that maximizing (13.25) in the case of many variable parameters may be difficult and extremely expensive computationally (this was not a problem in the previously mentioned implementation of the model of stereo signals [21], which was based upon optimizations specific to the case of two channels only).

References

[1] S. Mallat, *A Wavelet Tour of Signal Processing*, 2nd ed., New York: Academic Press, 1999.

[2] L. Cohen, *Time-Frequency Analysis*, Upper Saddle River, NJ: Prentice Hall, 1995.

[3] W. J. Williams, "Recent Advances in Time-Frequency Representations: Some Theoretical Foundations," in *Time Frequency and Wavelets in Biomedical Signal Processing*, M. Akay, (ed.), IEEE Press Series in Biomedical Engineering, New York: IEEE press, 1997, pp. 3–44.

[4] G. Davis, "Adaptive Nonlinear Approximations," Ph.D. thesis, New York University, 1994, ftp://cs.nyu.edu/pub/wave/report/DissertationGDavis.ps.Z.

[5] D. Harel, *Algorithmic: The Spirit of Computing*, 2nd ed., Reading, MA: Addison-Wesley, 1992.

[6] S. Mallat and Z. Zhang, "Matching Pursuit with Time-Frequency Dictionaries," *IEEE Transactions on Signal Processing*, vol. 41, December 1993, pp. 3397–3415.

[7] S. Qian and D. Chen, "Signal Representation Using Adaptive Normalized Gaussian Functions," *Signal Processing*, vol. 36, March 1994, pp. 1–11.

[8] Y. Pati, R. Rezaiifar, and P. Krishnaprasad, "Orthogonal Matching Pursuit: Recursive Function Approximation with Applications to Wavelet Decomposition," *Conference Record of the Twenty-Seventh Asilomar Conference on Signals, Systems and Computers*, vol. 1, October 1993, pp. 40–44.

[9] C. C. Jouny, P. J. Franaszczuk, and G. K. Bergey, "Characterization of Epileptic Seizure Dynamics Using Gabor Atom Density," *Clinical Neurophysiology*, vol. 114, 2003, pp. 426–437.

[10] R. Neff and A. Zakhor, "Modulus Quantization for Matching Pursuit Video Coding," *IEEE Transactions on Circuits and Systems for Video Technology*, vol. 10, no. 6, January 2000, pp. 13–26.

[11] C. de Vleeschouwer and A. Zakhor, "In-Loop Atom Modulus Quantization for Matching Pursuit and Its Application to Video Coding," *IEEE Transactions on Image Processing*, vol. 12, no. 10, October 2003, pp. 1226–1242.

[12] M. Goodwin, "Matching Pursuit with Damped Sinusoids," *Proc. ICASSP '97*, Munich, 1997, pp. 2037–2040.

[13] D. Ircha and P. J. Durka, "mp4 Software for Unbiased Matching Pursuit with Gabor Dictionaries," http://eeg.pl/Members/durka/Software.2004-02-20.5632, 2004.

[14] M. Barwiński, "Product-Based Metric for Gabor Functions and Its Implications for the Matching Pursuit Algorithm," M.S. thesis, Warsaw University, Institute of Experimental Physics, 2004, http://eeg.pl/Members/mbarwinski/Article.2004-09-21.0153.

[15] P. J. Durka, D. Ircha, and K. J. Blinowska, "Stochastic Time-Frequency Dictionaries for Matching Pursuit," *IEEE Transactions on Signal Processing*, vol. 49, no. 3, March 2001, pp. 507–510.

[16] K. J. Blinowska and P. J. Durka, "Unbiased High Resolution Method of EEG Analysis in Time-Frequency Space," *Acta Neurobiologiae Experimentalis*, vol. 61, 2001, pp. 157–174.

[17] R. A. DeVore and V. N. Temlyakov, "Some Remarks on Greedy Algorithms," *Advances in Computational Mathematics*, vol. 5, 1996, pp. 173–187.

[18] S. S. Chen, D. L. Donoho, and M. A. Saunders, "Atomic Decomposition by Basis Pursuit," *SIAM Review*, vol. 43, no. 1, 2001, pp. 129–159.

[19] S. Jaggi, et al., "High Resolution Pursuit for Feature Extraction," *LIDS Technical Reports*, number LIDS-P-2371, Laboratory for Information and Decision Systems, MIT, 1996.

[20] R. Gribonval, et al., "Sound Signals Decomposition Using a High Resolution Matching Pursuit," *Proc. Int. Computer Music Conf. (ICMC'96)*, August 1996, pp. 293–296.

[21] R. Gribonval, "Sparse Decomposition of Stereo Signals with Matching Pursuit and Application to Blind Separation of More Than Two Sources from a Stereo Mixture," *Acoustics, Speech, and Signal Processing, Proceedings of ICASSP '02*, Orlando, FL, vol. 3, May 2002, pp. 3057–3060.

[22] P. J. Durka, et al., "Multichannel Matching Pursuit and EEG Inverse Solutions," *Journal of Neuroscience Methods*, vol. 148, no. 1, 2005, pp. 49–59.

[23] D. Studer, U. Hoffmann, and T. Koenig, "From EEG Dependency Multichannel Matching Pursuit to Sparse Topographic Decomposition," *Journal of Neuroscience Methods*, vol. 153, 2006, pp. 261–275.

[24] R. Gribonval, "Piecewise Linear Source Separation," *Proc. SPIE 03*, San Diego, CA, August 2003.

[25] A. Matysiak, et al., "Time-Frequency-Space Localization of Epileptic EEG Oscillations," *Acta Neurobiologiae Experimentalis*, vol. 65, 2005, pp. 435–442.

[26] C. Tallon-Baudry, et al., "Stimulus Specificity of Phase-Locked and Non-Phase-Locked 40 Hz Visual Responses in Human," *The Journal of Neuroscience*, vol. 16, no. 13, 1996, pp. 4240–4249.

[27] A. Delorme and Scott Makeig, "EEGLAB: An Open Source Toolbox for Analysis of Single-Trial EEG Dynamics Including Independent Component Analysis," *Journal of Neuroscience Methods*, vol. 134, 2004, pp. 9–21.

Chapter 14

Implementation: Details and Tricks

This chapter describes some mathematical and programming tricks, necessary in real-world implementations of the matching pursuit algorithm.

Description of the MP algorithm is simple: *in each iteration we choose the function that gives the largest product with the signal.* Interpreted directly, this would imply that in *each* iteration we have to calculate the products of *all* the functions from the dictionary with the current residuum left from previous iterations. However, high-resolution approximations explored in this book require large dictionaries, so direct calculations of all the products in each step would result in prohibitive execution times.

Fortunately, several tricks can be employed in the implementations. We will concentrate upon two mathematical observations, which contribute the most significant computational gain in this context. Product update formula (Section 14.2) is specific to the MP algorithm; optimal phase selection (Section 14.1) is derived for Gabor functions. Section 14.3 exemplifies some of the numerical techniques that can be employed in this context.

In spite of these significant optimizations, computation cost of MP still grows significantly with the size of the dictionary and the number of iterations. Therefore, the most important gains can be achieved by adequate adjustment of the size (density) of the dictionary and the number of waveforms in MP expansion (regulated by the stopping criterion), in relation to requirements of particular applications. Dictionary density is discussed in Sections 7.1 and 13.8, and stopping criteria in Sections 7.2 and 13.7.

14.1 OPTIMAL PHASE OF A GABOR FUNCTION

Unfortunately, the only known way of finding parameters $\gamma_n = (u_n, \omega_n, s_n, \phi_n)$ of the function g_{γ_n}, which gives the largest product with the signal x (or the residuum $R^n x$), is the brute force approach, through calculating *all* the products $\langle x, g_{\gamma_i} \rangle$. *Fortunately*, this applies only to u, ω, and s. For a Gabor function of fixed u_i, ω_i, and s_i, we can easily find the unique phase $\phi_{\max}$ for which the product $\langle x, g_{(u_i, \omega_i, s_i, \phi_{\max})} \rangle$ will be maximum [1, 2]. Therefore, for the construction of the dictionary we need to sample only time and frequency centers and width, and avoid sampling the phase parameter. In the following, we will find an explicit formula for the phase $\phi_{\max}$, that maximizes the product of signal x with Gabor function of given time position u, frequency ω, and scale s.

Let us recall from Section 13.8 the formula (13.16) of a real Gabor function:

$$g_\gamma(t) = K(\gamma) e^{-\pi \left(\frac{t-u}{s}\right)^2} \cos\left(\omega(t-u) + \phi\right).$$

γ denotes the set of parameters $\gamma = \{u, s, \omega, \phi\}$ and $K(\gamma)$ is such that $||g_\gamma|| = 1$. Writing $K(\gamma)$ explicitly gives

$$g_{(\gamma)}(t) = \frac{e^{-\pi \left(\frac{t-u}{s}\right)^2} \cos\left(\omega(t-u) + \phi\right)}{||e^{-\pi \left(\frac{t-u}{s}\right)^2} \cos\left(\omega(t-u) + \phi\right)||} \tag{14.1}$$

Phase shift ϕ can be also expressed as a superposition of two orthogonal oscillations $\cos\left(\omega(t-u) + \phi\right)$ and $\sin\left(\omega(t-u) + \phi\right)$. We define

$$\begin{aligned} C &= e^{-\pi \left(\frac{t-u}{s}\right)^2} \cos\left(\omega(t-u)\right) \\ S &= e^{-\pi \left(\frac{t-u}{s}\right)^2} \sin\left(\omega(t-u)\right) \end{aligned} \tag{14.2}$$

and, using the trigonometric identity

$$\cos(\alpha + \phi) = \cos\alpha \cos\phi - \sin\alpha \sin\phi, \tag{14.3}$$

we write the Gabor function (14.1) as

$$g_\gamma(t) = \frac{C \cos\phi - S \sin\phi}{||C \cos\phi - S \sin\phi||} \tag{14.4}$$

Using $||x||^2 = \langle x, x \rangle$, and the orthogonality of C and S defined in (14.2) ($\langle C, S \rangle = 0$), we write the product of Gabor function defined as (14.4) with the signal x as

$$\langle x, g_\gamma \rangle = \frac{\langle x, C \rangle \cos\phi - \langle x, S \rangle \sin\phi}{\|C\cos\phi - S\sin\phi\|} = \frac{\langle x, C \rangle - \langle x, S \rangle \tan\phi}{\sqrt{\langle C, C \rangle + \langle S, S \rangle \tan^2\phi}} \tag{14.5}$$

We are looking for the maximum absolute value of this product. For the sake of simplicity we will maximize $\langle x, g_\gamma \rangle^2$ instead of $|\langle x, g_\gamma \rangle|$. Denoting $v = \tan\phi$

$$\langle x, g_\gamma \rangle^2 = \frac{(\langle x, C \rangle - \langle x, S \rangle v)^2}{\langle C, C \rangle + \langle S, S \rangle v^2} \tag{14.6}$$

To find v which maximizes (14.6), we look for zeros of the derivative:

$$\frac{\partial}{\partial v}\langle x, g_\gamma \rangle^2 = \frac{\partial}{\partial v}\, \frac{\langle x, C \rangle^2 + \langle x, S \rangle^2 v^2 - 2\langle x, C \rangle \langle x, S \rangle v}{\langle C, C \rangle + \langle S, S \rangle\, v^2} =$$

$$2\frac{\langle x, C \rangle \langle x, S \rangle \langle S, S \rangle v^2 + \left(\langle x, S \rangle^2 \langle C, C \rangle - \langle x, C \rangle^2 \langle S, S \rangle\right) v - \langle x, C \rangle \langle x, S \rangle \langle C, C \rangle}{\left(\langle C, C \rangle + \langle S, S \rangle\, v^2\right)^2}$$

Solving the quadratic equation in the nominator we get two roots:

$$v_1 = \frac{\langle x, C \rangle}{\langle x, S \rangle}, \qquad v_2 = -\frac{\langle x, S \rangle \langle C, C \rangle}{\langle x, C \rangle \langle S, S \rangle}$$

Substituting these values for $\tan\phi$ in (14.5) we get

$$\langle x, g_\gamma \rangle|_{v=v_1} = 0$$

$$\langle x, g_\gamma \rangle|_{v=v_2} = \frac{\langle x, C \rangle + \frac{\langle x, S \rangle^2 \langle C, C \rangle}{\langle x, C \rangle \langle S, S \rangle}}{\sqrt{\langle C, C \rangle + \frac{\langle x, S \rangle^2 \langle C, C \rangle^2}{\langle x, C \rangle^2 \langle S, S \rangle}}}$$

Obviously, for v_1 the square of the product is minimum (zero), so the other extremum is a maximum in v_2. Therefore, the phase ϕ that maximizes $\langle x, g_\gamma \rangle^2$ is given by

$$\phi_{\max} = \arctan \frac{\langle x, S \rangle / \langle S, S \rangle}{\langle x, C \rangle / \langle C, C \rangle} \tag{14.7}$$

and the maximum value of the product is

$$\langle x, g_\gamma \rangle_{\max} = \frac{\langle x, C \rangle^2 / \langle C, C \rangle + \langle x, S \rangle^2 / \langle S, S \rangle}{\sqrt{\langle x, C \rangle^2 / \langle C, C \rangle + \langle x, S \rangle^2 / \langle S, S \rangle}} \tag{14.8}$$

14.2 PRODUCT UPDATE FORMULA

In the nth iteration of MP we choose the atom g_{γ_n} that gives maximum $\langle R^n x, g_{\gamma_n}\rangle$. Let us recall part of (13.7):

$$R^n x = \langle R^n x, g_{\gamma_n}\rangle g_{\gamma_n} + R^{n+1}x$$

Taking the product of both sides with g_{γ_i}—a candidate for selection in the next iteration—and moving $\langle R^{n+1}x\rangle$ to the left, we get

$$\langle R^{n+1}x, g_{\gamma_i}\rangle = \langle R^n x, g_{\gamma_i}\rangle - \langle R^n x, g_{\gamma_n}\rangle\langle g_{\gamma_n}, g_{\gamma_i}\rangle \tag{14.9}$$

This equation expresses the product of a dictionary function g_{γ_i} with the residuum in step $n+1$ using two products, which were already calculated in the previous iteration—$\langle R^n x, g_{\gamma_i}\rangle$ and $\langle R^n x, g_{\gamma_n}\rangle$—and a product of two functions from the dictionary—$\langle g_{\gamma_n}, g_{\gamma_i}\rangle$. Therefore, the only thing that remains to be computed is a product of two known functions. This fact can be employed to significantly accelerate all iterations of MP except for the first one (e.g., using analytical formulae for these products).

Inner product of continuous Gabor functions can be expressed in terms of elementary functions (see [2, 3]). Unfortunately, it does not reflect with enough accuracy the numerical value of the product of two discrete vectors, representing sampled versions of the same Gabor functions. Exact formula for the product of the latter involves theta functions, which can be approximated by relatively fast converging series [3]. The software package "mpp" [4] implements a different approach, based upon the assumption that the signal outside the measured window is periodic. Formulae for this case are given in [5].

Apart from the actual way of calculating the product of two Gabors, we can a priori avoid calculations of these products, which will be close to zero (e.g., Gabors with narrow time support and distant time centers).

14.3 SIN, COS, AND EXP: FAST CALCULATIONS AND TABLES

In spite of the trick from the previous section, still—at least in the first iteration—we need to compute the "plain" inner products of the signal with Gabor functions. Using the result from Section 14.1, of all the phases ϕ in (13.16) we calculate products only for $\phi = 0$ and $\phi = \frac{\pi}{2}$.

Surprisingly, the most expensive[1] part is not the actual calculation of the inner products, but the generation of discrete vectors of samples from Equation (13.16), which contains cosine and exponent. Compilers usually approximate these functions by high-order polynomials. Although contemporary CPUs may implement directly some special functions, they will still be much more expensive to compute than basic additions or multiplications. Therefore, avoiding explicit calls of these functions may result in significant acceleration.[2] In the following we show (after [7]) how to fill in a vector with values of sines and cosines for equally spaced arguments using only one call of these functions.

Since the time t in (13.16) in the actual computations is discrete, the trick is to compute $\sin(\omega(t+1))$ knowing $\sin(\omega t)$. Using the trigonometric identity (14.3) with its corresponding form for the sine function, we get

$$\sin(\omega(t+1)) = \sin(\omega t + \omega) = \cos(\omega t)\sin(\omega) + \sin(\omega t)\cos(\omega) \tag{14.10}$$

$$\cos(\omega(t+1)) = \cos(\omega t + \omega) = \cos(\omega t)\cos(\omega) - \sin(\omega t)\sin(\omega) \tag{14.11}$$

We start with $t = 0$, setting $\cos(0) = 1$ and $\sin(0) = 0$, and computing constants $\cos(\omega)$ and $\sin(\omega)$. Values of (14.10) and (14.11) for subsequent t can be filled in a recursive way, using the computed $\cos(\omega)$ and $\sin(\omega)$ and taking as $\sin(\omega t)$ and $\cos(\omega t)$ values from the previous steps.

A similar approach can accelerate computation of the factors $e^{-\alpha t^2}$ present in (13.16):

$$e^{-\alpha(t+1)^2} = e^{-\alpha t^2 - 2\alpha t - \alpha} = e^{-\alpha t^2} e^{-2\alpha t} e^{-\alpha} \tag{14.12}$$

To compute (14.12) we need $e^{-\alpha t^2}$ from the previous iteration, constant $e^{-\alpha}$ independent of t, and $e^{-2\alpha t}$. The last factor can be updated in each iteration at a cost of one multiplication: to get $e^{-2\alpha(t+1)}$ from $e^{-2\alpha t}$ we multiply it by a precomputed constant $e^{-2\alpha}$.

In all these cases we also take into account the symmetries $\sin(-x) = -\sin(x)$, $\cos(-x) = \cos(x)$, and $e^{-(-x)^2} = e^{-x^2}$ to double the savings. Values of these vectors can be stored in memory for subsequent calculations of Gabor vectors (13.16) with different combinations of sin/cos and exp, but only if we restrict the discretization of parameters to some integer grid, for example:

$$u = 1 \ldots N, \quad \omega = (1 \ldots N)\pi/N, \quad s = 1 \ldots N \tag{14.13}$$

1 In terms of computation times.

2 Used together with tabularization, it accelerated the MP implementation [6] by over an order of magnitude.

References

[1] S. E. Ferrando, L. A. Kolasa, and N. Kovačević, "A Flexible Implementation of Matching Pursuit for Gabor Functions on the Interval," *ACM Transactions on Mathematical Software (TOMS)*, vol. 28, 2002, pp. 337–353.

[2] M. Barwiński, "Product-Based Metric for Gabor Functions and Its Implications for the Matching Pursuit Algorithm," M.S. thesis, Warsaw University, Institute of Experimental Physics, 2004, http://eeg.pl/Members/mbarwinski/Article.2004-09-21.0153.

[3] S. E. Ferrando, et al., "Probabilistic Matching Pursuit with Gabor Dictionaries," *Signal Processing*, vol. 80, no. 10, 2000, pp. 2099–2120.

[4] S. Mallat and Z. Zhang, "Matching Pursuit Software Package (mpp)," 1993, ftp://cs.nyu.edu/pub/wave/software/mpp.tar.Z.

[5] S. Mallat and Z. Zhang, "Matching Pursuit with Time-Frequency Dictionaries," *IEEE Transactions on Signal Processing*, vol. 41, December 1993, pp. 3397–3415.

[6] D. Ircha and P. J. Durka, "mp4 Software for Unbiased Matching Pursuit with Gabor Dictionaries," http://eeg.pl/Members/durka/Software.2004-02-20.5632, 2004.

[7] D. Ircha, "Reprezentacje sygnałów w redundantnych zbiorach funkcji," M.S. thesis, Warsaw University, Institute of Experimental Physics, 1997.

Chapter 15

Statistical Significance of Changes in the Time-Frequency Plane

This chapter presents technical and mathematical details of the procedure of assessing the statistical significance of the even-related signal energy changes in the time-frequency plane.

15.1 REFERENCE EPOCH

A typical ERD/ERS experiment (Chapter 10) collects N trials. Each trial consists of a period of the signal prior to the event—a reference period t_{ref} that we assume is unaffected by the event—and an event period t_{ev}, the period of signal during which the investigated event-related changes may occur. Properties of the signal in the reference epoch should reflect the "normal" state of the signal, in the sense that the measured changes will be relative to these properties.

Strict assumption of stationarity of the signals in the reference epoch would make an elegant derivation of the applied statistics: the repetitions could be then treated as realizations of an ergodic process. Indeed, epochs of EEG up to 10-seconds duration (recorded under constant behavioral conditions) are usually considered stationary [1]. However, the assumption of "constant behavioral conditions" can probably be challenged in some cases. We cannot test this assumption directly, since the usual length of the reference epoch is too short for a standard test of signal stationarity.[1] Nevertheless, bootstrapping the available data across the indexes corresponding to time and repetition (trial number) simultaneously does not require a strict assumption of ergodicity from the purely statistical point of view. But we must be aware that this fact does not diminish our responsibility in the choice of the reference epoch, which in general should be long enough to represent the "reference" properties of the signal to which the changes will be related, and at the same time it should be distant enough from both the beginning of the recorded epoch (to avoid the influence of border conditions) and the investigated phenomenon (to not include some event-related properties in the reference).

15.2 RESOLUTION ELEMENTS

For each of the N trials ($n = 1, \ldots, N$) we estimate the time-frequency energy density $E_n(t, f)$ at the finest possible grid, as in Plate 5. However, assessment of the statistical significance of changes at given time-frequency coordinates is performed at a lower resolution, in time-frequency boxes $\Delta t \times \Delta f$.

Time-frequency resolution of the signal's energy density estimate depends on a multitude of factors, which are even more complicated in the case of the averages computed for N trials. A general lower bound is given by the uncertainty principle [3], which states that the product of the time and frequency variances exceeds $\frac{1}{16\pi^2}$:

$$\sigma_t^2 \sigma_f^2 \geq \frac{1}{16\pi^2} \tag{15.1}$$

Here the frequency f is defined as inverse of the period (Hz). For the angular frequency ω, (15.1) would be: $\sigma_t^2 \sigma_\omega^2 \geq \frac{1}{4}$. It can be proved that equality in these equations is achieved by complex Gabor functions; other functions give higher values of this product [4]. Since the time and frequency spreads are proportional to the square root of the corresponding variances, a minimum of their product reaches $\frac{1}{4\pi}$.

However, attempts to estimate the statistical significance in resels of area as small as given by (15.1) result in detection of isolated changes, that are not stable

1 Standard test for stationarity relies on dividing the questioned epoch into subepochs of the length exceeding the period of the lowest frequency present in the signal, and then applying a nonparametric test (e.g., sign test) to statistical descriptors of these subepochs [2]. The usual length of the reference epoch does not exceed seconds, so considering the presence of low EEG frequencies (order of few hertz), we would have too few subepochs for a reasonable application of a low-power nonparametric test.

in respect to varying other parameters of the procedure. To decrease this noise, we fixed the area of resels at $\frac{1}{2}$, which at least has certain statistical justification: standard, generally used sampling of the spectrogram gives $\frac{1}{2}$ as the product of the localization in time (window length) and in frequency (interval between estimated frequencies). This sampling is based upon statistically optimal properties, namely independent samples for a periodogram of a Gaussian random process [5]; other values of this parameter can of course be considered in practical applications.

In such a way we achieve the necessary discretization of the time-frequency plane into resels $r(i,j)$, centered in (t_i, f_j), with dimensions $\Delta t \times \Delta f$. MP decomposition (13.11) generates a continuous map of the energy density (13.23) for each single trial (index tr) of an experiment. From this decomposition a discrete map must be calculated with a finite resolution. The simplest solution is to sum for each resel the values of all the functions from the expansion (13.11) in the center of each resel (t_i, f_j):

$$E_{\mathrm{tr}}(t_i, f_j) = \sum_n | < R^n s,\ g_{\gamma_n} > |^2\ \mathcal{W}g_{\gamma_n}(t_i, f_j) \tag{15.2}$$

However, for certain structures or relatively large resels, (15.2) may not be representative for the amount of energy contained within its boundaries. Therefore we use the exact solution, obtained by integrating, for each resel, the power of all the functions from expansion (13.11) within the ranges corresponding to the resel's boundaries:

$$E_{\mathrm{tr}}(i,j) = E_{\mathrm{tr}}(t_i, f_j) = \sum_n | < R^n f, g_{\gamma_n} > |^2 \int_{t_i-\frac{\Delta t}{2}}^{t_i+\frac{\Delta t}{2}} \int_{f_j-\frac{\Delta f}{2}}^{f_j+\frac{\Delta f}{2}} \mathcal{W}g_{\gamma_n}(t, f)dtdf \tag{15.3}$$

Integral in this equation has no analytical solution—it has to be calculated numerically.

15.3 STATISTICS

To express the change of the mean (across the trials) energy in the resel (i,j), in relation to the mean (across the trials and resels in the same frequency contained in the reference epoch) energy in the reference period, we can use the t statistics:

$$t_{i,j} = \frac{\overline{E_{\text{ref}}(\cdot, j)} - \overline{E(i,j)}}{s_\Delta} \tag{15.4}$$

where $\overline{E(i,j)} = \frac{1}{N}\sum_{\text{tr}=1}^{N} E_{\text{tr}}(i,j)$ denotes mean energy in resel (i,j), $E_{\text{ref}}(\cdot, j)$ relates to the mean energy in the reference period for frequency f_j, and s_Δ is the pooled variance of energy in the reference epoch and in the investigated resel. Such statistics can be used for both parametric and nonparametric tests: it is pivotal for normally distributed data, and in other cases it is asymptotically pivotal [6].

15.4 RESAMPLING

If we cannot assume the energies, calculated in resels, to be distributed normally, we estimate the distribution of statistics t (15.4) by bootstrapping $E_{\text{tr}}(i,j)$ in the reference epoch, separately for each frequency j. That is:

1. From the energies $E_{\text{tr}}(i,j)$ in the reference epoch ($i \in t_{\text{ref}}$), draw with replacement two samples: A of size N, and B of size $N \cdot N_{\text{ref}}$, where N is the number of experiment trials, and N_{ref} is the number of resels in the reference period.
2. Treating sample A as representing a resel under hypothesis of no change, and sample B as the reference, statistics $t_{\cdot,j}$ from (15.4).
3. Repeat steps 1 and 2 N_{rep} times.

The set of computed values $t_{\cdot,j}$ approximates the distribution $T_{\text{resamp}}(j)$ at frequency j. For each resel (i,j) the actual value of (15.4) is compared to this distribution:

$$p(i,j) = 2\min\left\{P\left(T_{\text{resamp}}(j) \geq t(i,j)\right), 1 - P\left(T_{\text{resamp}}(j) \geq t(i,j)\right)\right\} \tag{15.5}$$

yielding two-sided $p(i,j)$ for the null hypothesis of no energy change. The relative error of p is (see [7])

$$err = \frac{\sigma_p}{p} = \sqrt{\frac{(1-p)}{pN_{\text{rep}}}} \tag{15.6}$$

As in most of the resampling methods, this algorithm is computationally intensive. Due to the widespread availability of computing resources, it causes no problems in most of the standard applications. However, corrections for multiple comparisons imply very low effective critical values of the probabilities needed to reject the null hypothesis. For the analysis presented in this book, the FDR adjustments gave critical values of the order of 10^{-4}. If we set this for p in (15.6), we obtain a minimum of $N_{\text{rep}} = 10^6$ resampling repetitions to achieve 10% relative error for the values $p(i, j)$.

15.5 PARAMETRIC TESTS

Computational complexity of the procedure from the previous section turns our attention back to the classical methods. However, in order to apply parametric tests, we need to transform $E_{\text{tr}}(i, j)$ in such a way that the resulting variable will have a normal distribution. As proven in [8], in the investigated EEG and ECoG data, this was possible using the Box-Cox transformation [9], which is actually a family of power transformations:

$$BC(x, \lambda) = \begin{cases} \frac{x^{\lambda}-1}{\lambda} & if \quad \lambda \neq 0 \\ \log(x) & if \quad \lambda = 0 \end{cases} \tag{15.7}$$

In each frequency j the λ parameter is optimized by maximization of log-likelihood function in the reference period:

$$\lambda_{\text{opt}}^{j} = \max_{\lambda} \{LLF(\lambda)\} = \max_{\lambda} \left\{ -\frac{m}{2} \log \sigma^2_{BC(x,\lambda)} + (\lambda - 1) \sum_{k=1}^{m} \log x_k \right\} \tag{15.8}$$

where m is the length of data x, $x_k \in \{E_n(i, j) : i \in t_{\text{ref}}, n = 1, \ldots, N\}$. The optimal λ_{opt}^{j} is then used to transform all the resels in frequency j.

If, after this transformation, the distribution of energies is approximately normal, we can avoid the resampling procedures outlined in the previous section and use the parametric t-test. In this approach we also use the formula (15.4), but in this case we assume that $t(i, j)$ conforms to the Student's t-distribution with $f = N + N \cdot N_{\text{ref}} - 2$ degrees of freedom.

15.6 CORRECTION FOR MULTIPLE COMPARISONS

All of these statistical tests were applied to energies in each resel separately. However, the very notion of the test's confidence level reflects the possibility of falsely rejecting the null hypothesis. For example, a confidence level of 5% means that it may happen in approximately 1 in 20 cases. If we evaluate many such tests, we are very likely to obtain many such false rejections. This issue is known in statistics as the issue of multiple comparisons, and there are several ways to deal with it properly.

The most straightforward approach is the so-called Bonferroni adjustment, which relies on dividing the confidence level of each test by the total number of performed tests. In most cases, it is definitely too conservative. Following [10], we employ a procedure assessing the False Discovery Rate (FDR, proposed in [11]). The FDR is the ratio of the number of falsely rejected null hypotheses (m_0) to the number of all rejected null hypotheses (m). In our case, if we control the FDR at a level $q = 0.05$ we know that among resels, declared as revealing significant changes of energy, at most 5% are declared so falsely (false discoveries). Reference [11] proves that the following procedure controls the FDR at the level q:

1. Order the achieved significance levels p_i, approximated in the previous section for all the resels separately, in an ascending series: $p_1 \leq p_2 \leq \cdots \leq p_m$
2. Find

$$k = \max\{i : p_i \leq \frac{i}{m \sum_{j=1}^{m} \frac{1}{j}} q\} \tag{15.9}$$

3. Reject all hypotheses for which $p \leq p_k$ (p_k is the effective significance level).

Resels $r(i, j)$ are marked significant if the null hypothesis $H_0^{i,j}$ can be rejected using the significance level p_k for the probabilities $p(i, j)$ of the null hypothesis.

Finally, within the boundaries of the area of these significant resels, the map of ERD/ERS values (as defined in [12]) is displayed:

$$\text{ERD/ERS}(t, f) = \frac{\overline{E(t, f)} - \overline{E_{\text{ref}}(\cdot, f)}}{\overline{E_{\text{ref}}(\cdot, f)}} \tag{15.10}$$

where $\overline{E_{\text{ref}}(\cdot, f)}$ and $\overline{E(t, f)}$ are average defined as those in (15.4), but here t_i, f_j refer to the maximum resolution of the time-frequency estimate rather than resels chosen in Section 15.2.

References

[1] E. Niedermayer and F. Lopes Da Silva, *Electroencephalography: Basic Principles, Clinical Applications and Related Fields*, 4th ed., Baltimore, MD: Williams & Wilkins, 1999.

[2] J. S. Bendat and A. G. Piersol, *Random Data: Analysis and Measurement Procedures*, New York: John Wiley & Sons, 1971.

[3] L. Cohen, *Time-Frequency Analysis*, Upper Saddle River, NJ: Prentice Hall, 1995.

[4] S. Mallat, *A Wavelet Tour of Signal Processing*, 2nd ed., New York: Academic Press, 1999.

[5] M. B. Priestley, *Spectral Analysis and Time Series*, New York: Academic Press, 1981.

[6] P. H. Westfall and S. S. Young, *Resampling-Based Multiple Testing*, New York: John Wiley & Sons, 1993.

[7] B. Efron and R. J. Tibshirani, *An Introduction to the Bootstrap*, London: Chapman & Hall, 1993.

[8] J. Żygierewicz, et al., "Computationally Efficient Approaches to Calculating Significant ERD/ERS Changes in the Time-Frequency Plane," *Journal of Neuroscience Methods*, vol. 145, no. 1–2, 2005, pp. 267–276.

[9] G. E. P. Box and D. R. Cox, "An Analysis of Transformations," *Journal of the Royal Statistical Society*, vol. 2, 1964, pp. 211–252.

[10] P. J. Durka, et. al., "On the Statistical Significance of Event-Related EEG Desynchronization and Synchronization in the Time-Frequency Plane," *IEEE Transactions on Biomedical Engineering*, vol. 51, 2004, pp. 1167–1175.

[11] Y. Benjamini and Y. Yekutieli, "The Control of the False Discovery Rate Under Dependency," *Ann. Stat.*, vol. 29, 2001, pp. 1165–1188.

[12] G. Pfurtscheller, "EEG Event-Related Desynchronization (ERD) and Event-Related Synchronization (ERS)," in *Electroencephalography: Basic Principles, Clinical Applications and Related Fields*, 4th ed., E. Niedermayer and F. Lopes Da Silva, (eds.), Baltimore, MD: Williams & Wilkins, 1999, pp. 958–965.

About the Author

Piotr J. Durka received an M.Sc. and a Ph.D. and habilitation in physics from the Warsaw University. His views on the mission of a physicist in biomedical sciences are coherent with Richard Feynman's speech on cargo cult science, Jon Clearbout's notion of reproducible research, and the Occam's Razor.

In 1995 Dr. Durka introduced matching pursuit to biomedical signal analysis; these early studies were among the first real-world applications of adaptive time-frequency approximations. After a decade of continued work, subsequent applications reached the critical volume needed to support his thesis about possible unification in the field of EEG analysis. In 2004 he proposed SignalML (http://signalml.org), an elegant solution to the problem of incompatibility of digital formats used for storage of biomedical time series.

His other activities include being the president of award-winning software company Bitlab Ltd. (1994–1997), design of the EEG.pl neuroinformatics portal (2003), lectures on signal processing, statistics, and computer science, and writing three books. For a full list of research papers, software, and other information, see http://durka.info.

Index

Recent Related Titles from Artech House

Advanced Methods and Tools for ECG Data Analysis, Gari D. Clifford, Francisco Azuaje, and Patrick E. McSharry, editors

Biomolecular Computation for Bionanotechnology, Jian-Qin Liu and Katsunori Shimohara

Electrotherapeutic Devices: Principles, Design, and Applications, George D. O'Clock

Fundamentals and Applications of Microfluidics, Second Edition, Nam-Trung and Steven T. Wereley

Intelligent Systems Modeling and Decision Support in Bioengineering, Mahdi Mahfouf

Microfluidics for Biotechnology, Jean Berthier and Pascal Silberzan

Systems Bioinformatics: An Engineering Case-Based Approach, Gil Alterovitz and Marco R. Ramoni, editors

Text Mining for Biology and Biomedicine, Sophia Ananiadou and John McNaught, editors

For further information on these and other Artech House titles, including previously considered out-of-print books now available through our In-Print-Forever® (IPF®) program, contact:

Artech House
685 Canton Street
Norwood, MA 02062
Phone: 781-769-9750
Fax: 781-769-6334
e-mail: artech@artechhouse.com

Artech House
46 Gillingham Street
London SW1V 1AH UK
Phone: +44 (0)20 7596-8750
Fax: +44 (0)20 7630-0166
e-mail: artech-uk@artechhouse.com

Find us on the World Wide Web at: www.artechhouse.com